Flying Free

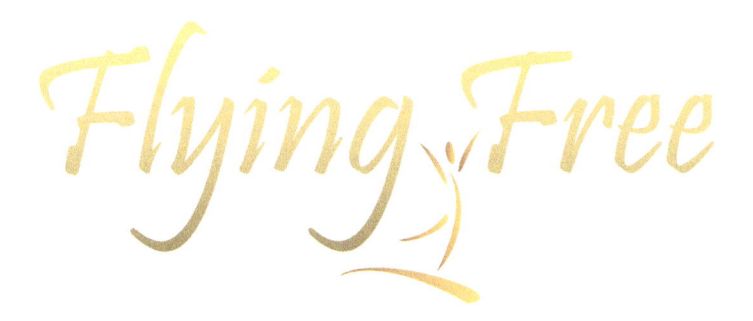

Powerful Journeys of those who DARE to LIVE!

Inspired within by
Jacinta McShane

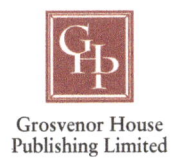

Grosvenor House
Publishing Limited

All rights reserved
Copyright © Jacinta McShane, 2015
www.centreoflivinghope.co.uk
hiddengifts@hotmail.co.uk

The right of Jacinta McShane to be identified as the author of this
work has been asserted in accordance with Section 78
of the Copyright, Designs and Patents Act 1988

The front cover image is copyright to Sergii Denysov

This book is published by
Grosvenor House Publishing Ltd
28-30 High Street, Guildford, Surrey, GU1 3EL.
www.grosvenorhousepublishing.co.uk

This book is sold subject to the conditions that it shall not, by way of
trade or otherwise, be lent, resold, hired out or otherwise circulated
without the author's or publisher's prior consent in any form of binding or
cover other than that in which it is published and
without a similar condition including this condition being imposed
on the subsequent purchaser.

A CIP record for this book
is available from the British Library

ISBN 978-1-78148-494-4

'Choosing to Thrive through Cancer'

To my son Josh
My wonder
You have your wings
Fly free my darling

Dedication

To my beautiful, 'still' friend Geraldine Dunn.

I first met Geraldine seventeen years ago when I enrolled for weekly Meditation classes locally. I remember feeling so proud of myself, being able to bring my three year old son with me as there was an on- site crèche. We connected almost immediately.

Geraldine became my lifeline as I went to theatre for cancer surgery several times years later. She stayed with me during my first biopsy, much to the annoyance of everyone else. She came with me down to theatre for surgery several times, even when she wasn't allowed. She was by my bedside when I woke up, whether at night or by day.

Holding my hand all the way, she affirmed with love and complete stillness: "Jacinta, you know that you are more than your body, don't you!" I didn't understand what she meant at the time, but somewhere deep inside I knew it was what I needed, without knowing why. Afterwards, she would be by my bedside smiling softly as I opened my eyes. I was amazed to realize that I had made it through and I was alive.

Geraldine was almost 70 and had lung cancer.

I now know without a doubt that I am so much more than my body. She gave me the greatest gift of all!

Bless You

Special angels (in human form of course) surround me as 'Flying Free' is born gently and divinely.

Elaine Ferguson: Little did I know that crossing paths with you at SPACE in St. Mary's Church in Aylesbury several years ago, and then meeting you again accidently in the street as an Aylesbury Chaplain, would draw us together in this spiritual way. Thank you for offering, unconditionally, to edit my manuscript and doing it so beautifully, diligently and quickly! "You made the whole task so much easier, Elaine; your advice was so valuable and just knowing you were always there, gave me the extra strength when I needed it. I don't think I could have let this book leave me without your encouragement."

Thrivers - a very special thank you to the remarkable, daring 'Thrivers' who are at the heart of this book: your amazing stories have inspired me on my own journey and moved me to write this book: "I feel blessed that you could share your challenges, vulnerabilities and triumphs with me so openly and allow me to bring them out into the light".

Bruce and Vicky Northey (missionaries in Mexico). Bless you both. You brought me to the divine light within, you loved us and brought us into your family. You gave us more than you will ever know.

Mrs Issels and the vocational Doctors of Issels Immuno-oncology – Bless you you for treating and healing all of me with hope, love and faith.

Simon Deere: Bless you for making the impossible possible and stepping forward into the brink.

Alison May: Bless you for walking with me where others fear to tread.

Waddesdon, Bucks: Bless the warm, embracing community of our home village of Waddesdon.

Profile

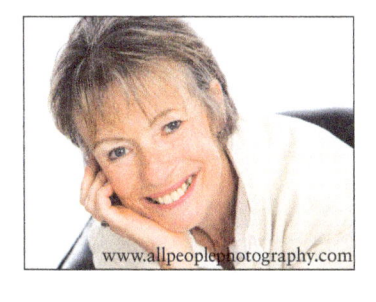

I never thought I would be alive today, never mind write a second book!

My own cancer journey over the past eleven years has opened up the world for me and given me life.

I have made choices I never thought I would, held beliefs I didn't know I had, turned inside out and didn't know I could! I feel I have been everywhere, here and abroad, exploring and receiving conventional and complementary treatment, speaking at various events, exchanging inspirational healing stories with many people, not just here in UK, but Ireland, Europe, USA, Australia, South Africa etc. As a result, I just have to share with you a little of the wonder, hope, love and healing that is out there.

It feels completely natural to write and facilitate this book as others' cherished, life-changing experiences of cancer gently unfold, flowing through me, through these pages as it is meant to be.

I am sure that being in the same boat enables me to write 'Flying Free' from the 'inside', as it were. This feels effortless, fearless, limitless and fulfilling, all at the same time. I feel truly privileged, guided and blessed.

Calling

Standing bare
atop this majestic peak
wrapped in love
I look back

Scrambling through deep dark undergrowth
resisting every step of the way
hands gripping tight
fingertips ablaze, white with strain
I hold on fiercely to what I have known

Yet a power greater than all
drawing me, guiding me
through this laden swamp of fear
to this moment
of light and clarity
ease and love
healing and vitality

**I choose this path
I hear your call!**

Contents

Dedications	v
Bless you	vii
Profile	ix
Forward!	xv
Opening	xvii
THE END	1
Al – "I have four cruises in me"	7
Michelle: "I never stopped being in awe of the beauty and majestic power of nature in all its glory".	13
Jay: "God, I thank you for this pain"	31
Iain: "If cancer is a messenger, it has an urgent message. If I can interpret that, I stand some chance of putting it right"	**49**
Gordon: "I am now flying and free of the chains that had been holding me down. Life is exciting"	67
Glenn: "I had to go forward from here"	95
Centre of Living Hope	**114**

CONTENTS

Marilyn: "My life so far had provided enough stressful experiences for ten lifetimes but gradually, one by one, I made peace with them all" — 117

Helen: "I always knew there was so much more!" — 137

Nina: "I have been training for this all my life" — 159

Pauline: "There is ALWAYS something to be thankful for" — 173

Claire: "Look up my darling, don't look back!" — 187

Jacinta (Author): "I needed cancer in my life to heal completely" — 207

THE BEGINNING — 217

Onward! — 220

All the little Advice — 221

References — 231

Celebrate Your Journey — 234

Yes to Life — 235

Hidden Gifts – A Preview — 237

Forward!

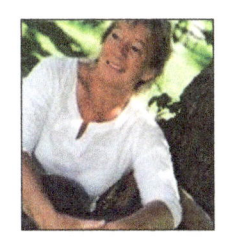

In February 2004, something extraordinary and unexpected happened that had an enormous impact on the rest of my life.

My very dear friend Jacinta asked me to accompany her to The Issels Immunotherapy Treatment Centre in Mexico to continue her healing treatment for Breast Cancer. We had already been through a lot together in our lives, me being present at the birth of her beautiful son Josh, and then attending hospital appointments after she first heard the debilitating news that she had breast cancer. It felt completely right that I should accompany her on this next stage of her healing, so without hesitation, I said "yes".

Issels is unique in its patient care, and from my research I knew that my very special friend was going to receive an extraordinary healing experience there, which was exactly what happened. Being witness to Jacinta finding God in her life, and letting go of all past trauma, was such a joy to witness. To see her find peace in her life was a true gift to observe and, I believe, the start to her true healing.

For me, it enabled me to experience miracles on every level: I began an education that has led me to where I am today. Beginning with a deep understanding of why an alkaline-based diet is important to help preventing cancer, to realising that the 'will' of a person to survive, is of the utmost importance, and finding an inner peace. My life has had its twists and turns since my trip to Issels, but I have always held my faith that out of something bad comes good. Even though at those times I couldn't see it, in each case this has been proven right. There is always a healing lesson to be learned through every choice we make.

It is gorgeous to watch my friend from afar, offering reassurance and healing to others through her love and compassion for humanity as a whole.

I will always be thankful to her for the true gift of love and understanding she has given me through her own divine healing. Thank you, Jacinta.

Claire Feltham

Opening

In a small healing room in Mexico back in 2007, people with all sorts of cancers enthuse about all the blessings in their lives. I listen in awe. I am floored to hear each person enthuse joyously about all their blessings, regardless of how ill they are. I cannot think of one blessing, but as the days blend into weeks, these blessings begin to pour out, uplifting, inspiring, strengthening us beyond ourselves!

This experience affected me deeply and gloriously. This lies at the heart of my first book: 'Hidden Gifts', my own healing story see Preview on Page 237.

Since then, my world has opened up even more. I feel I have been everywhere, exploring, engaging, experiencing, embracing, immersing, healing. I see a wonderful, uplifting, inspiring face of this disease, a face that does not come across in the media. It's my intention to redress this balance. I feel called to share this amazing spirit through the unique personal experiences of eleven outstanding individuals who invite you into their inspirited worlds. They are 'beyond' their cancers. They are 'beyond' themselves.

Crossing Paths
The remarkable people I have had the privilege to know are those living with cancer, families, missionaries and vocational doctors at The Issels Immunotherapy

Treatment Centre and The Oasis of Hope Hospital in Tijuana, Mexico, The Global Retreat Centre in Nuneham Courtney, Oxfordshire, The Breasts Friends' Cancer Support Group in Aylesbury, Bucks, The Pink Ladies' Cancer support group in my original home town of Derry, Northern Ireland, and The Hospice of St. Francis in Hertfordshire.

Thriving!

These wonderful, unassuming individuals do me the honour of sharing their truly living experiences and triumphs, flowing through these pages: from some thriving with cancer themselves; surviving, thriving relatives of those who have passed away, and my story of an unexpected friendship. I cannot, in all honesty, use the nondescript term: 'Cancer Patient', nor can I refer to these outstanding individuals as 'Cancer Survivors', limiting in itself: but 'Cancer Thrivers' who dare to live magnificently.

Connecting

Initially, I emailed some of the amazing individuals who have touched me, inviting them to share their personal story through the pages of 'Flying Free', giving them a broad outline of my book. I wanted to hear more about how cancer changed their lives and the lives of their loved ones, or rather, how they changed their lives through cancer for the better, practically, emotionally and most of all spiritually. As these remarkable individuals are scattered across the globe, I approached this in several different ways to ensure that all stories were in thrivers' own words: meeting up personally or by telephone, listening and recording their stories which I later transcribed, asking those living abroad to write their own stories and others who preferred to write their own.

Flowing Organically
I was keen to avoid limiting this process through deadlines, number of words, grammar etc. My intention has been for these stories to flow as organically as possible from heart and soul through the pages of this book with as little intervention as possible. Hence this book has taken as much time as it has needed to come together of its own volition, as it were. I wrote the opening and closing chapters, my own healing chapter on my unexpected friendship and brief comments at the beginning of each chapter of how each of these 'thrivers' touched me. Otherwise, the guts of this book are the special individuals themselves.

Emerging as 'Flying Free'
When I first thought of creating this book, about three years ago, I pictured the title as: 'Reach' with a powerful image of an arm with an outstretched hand bursting through the earth, straining very hard to reach the sunlight above which, in retrospect, was how I used to see cancer. My son commented that it sounded like the cover of a horror story. As time passed by, and as I listened more deeply, I changed. 'Reach' implying so much effort and pain, faded away and 'Flying Free' gently emerged.

Inspiring The Cover
Sitting in Prayers early one morning in hospital in Mexico five years ago, I heard one of the missionaries had been up during the night with a lady who was in a lot of pain. The next moment, as people slowly arrived,

this lady walked in, fully dressed with her hair tied back, smiling. Clearly suffering physically, she serenely read out a poem she had written during the night in the midst of her darkness. All I can remember of the poem is the lightness in the last line of each verse – reverberating gently again and again: '…. and I look out the window and the birds are flying across the sun'. '…and I look out the window and the birds are flying across the sun'. '…and I look out the window and the birds are flying across the sun', now inspiring the front cover.

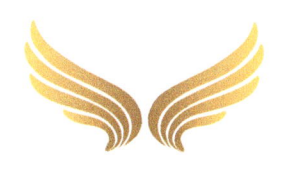

*"We may feel it is the end;
it is only the beginning!"*

The End

One minute we are going about our daily lives: taking the kids to school, driving to work, fixing the car, holding meetings, cooking dinner, washing up, reading bed-time stories, paying bills, going on holiday. The next instant, we are hit by cancer: endless hospital visits, operations, anaesthetics, medications, infusions, radiotherapy, chemotherapy, scans, x-rays, blood tests and more and more! Cancer has suddenly erupted and taken over our 'normal' lives. Everything has stopped. Everything has changed. *We may feel it is the end; it is only the beginning!*

When initially caught up in the gruelling grip and throes of cancer, it is almost impossible to imagine that life will ever be the same again. This is true, but what is also true, is that life can be better, lighter, more uplifting and empowering! 'Crisis' derived from the ancient Greek word 'crisis' means choice, a separating, a power of distinguishing. Some call it a turning-point.

Facing crisis gives us an 'unbelievable' opportunity to change, an 'unlikely' opportunity to heal deeply, whether we realize it or not. The choice is entirely in our hands and NOT in the hands of our doctors, families, friends, therapists or anyone else! It's up to each of us to decide if we truly want to heal, or coast along passively till we fade away. Even 'not making a choice' is in itself a choice. It is always our choice! That's the beauty, the responsibility and the wonderful power of it!

There are so many myths and assumptions about cancer, mostly coming from hearing about cancer through media and others' horror stories, myths like: I might get worse if I talk about it! My life is over; I will never cope; I can do this alone; I am going to die now! My life is in the doctors' hands! I have only got months to live! I must keep life going as normal; I will never get over this; life will never get any better; I will never heal! 'Flying Free' does not just dispel these myths, it blasts them out of the water removing the darkness of cancer, letting the light shine magnificently and showing us that this can be the beginning!

'Flying Free' gives you a glimpse of the true power and magnificence within us all, a power that surpasses us and a magnificence that outshines us all – glorious, glorious, glorious light!

As you read, allow yourself to fly from the depths of your being, as you immerse yourself in the joy, love and complete freedom within.

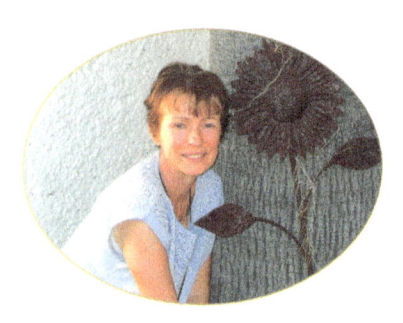

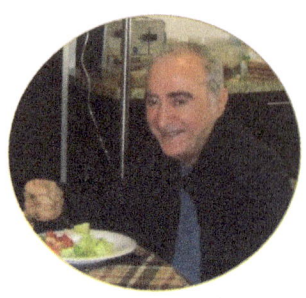

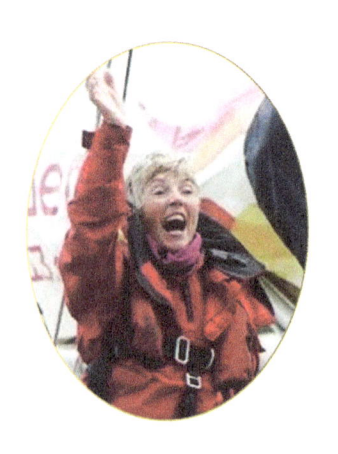

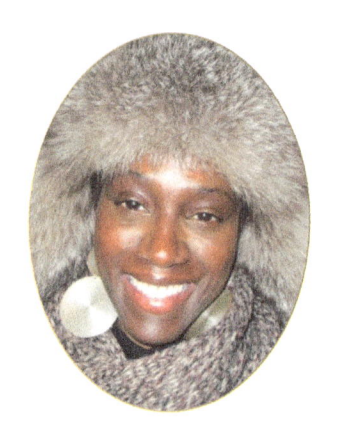

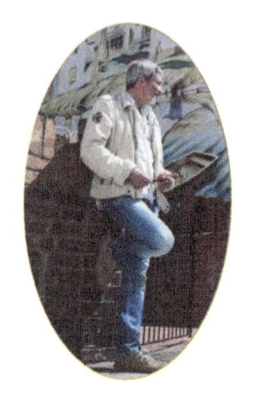

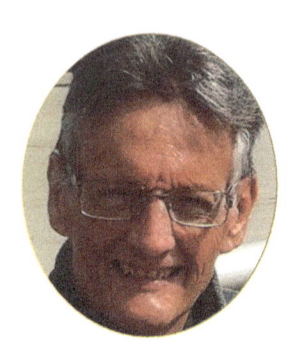

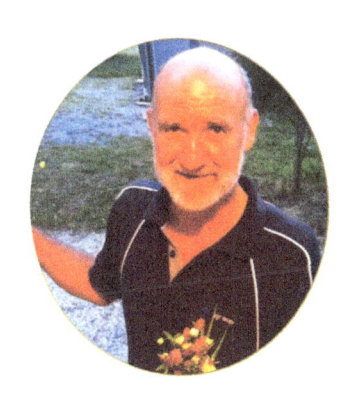

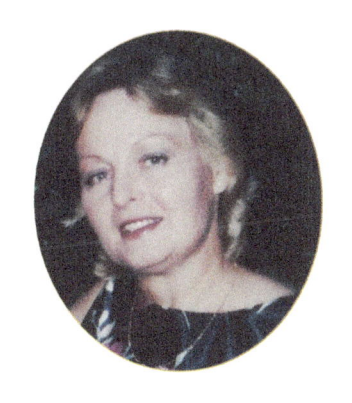

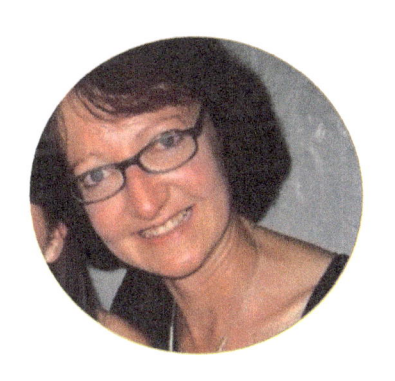

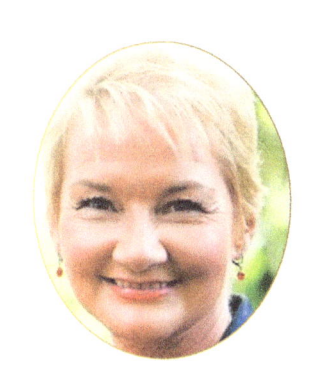

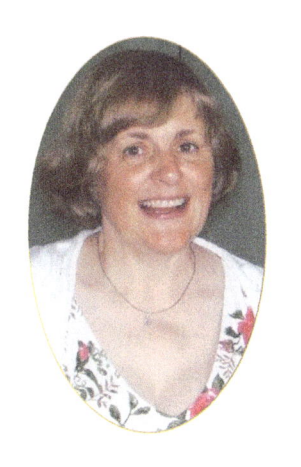

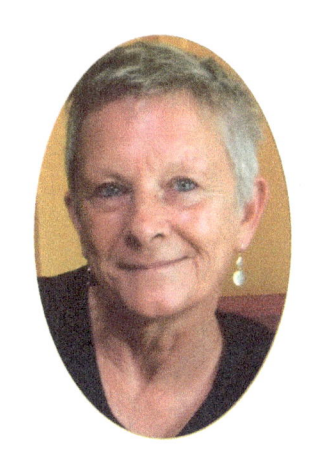

"I have four cruises in me now!"

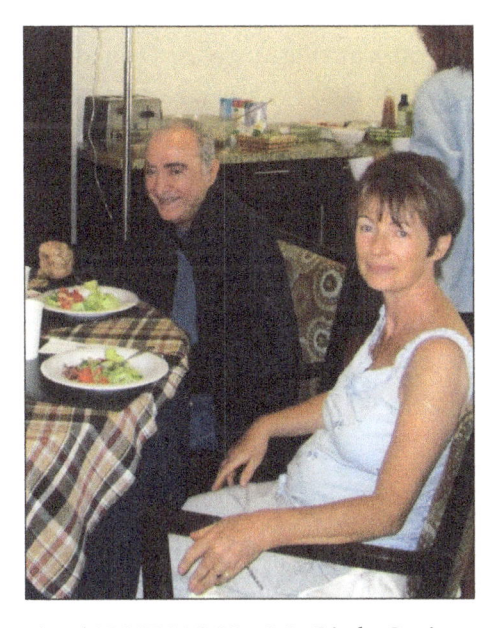

AL ANGELUCCI – My Little Cruiser

Here I share my own unexpected experience and beautiful connection with Al in Mexico.

I met Al for the first time when I joined him at the dining table in Oasis of Hope Hospital in Mexico.

He sat, head drooping, gazing forlornly into his full plate of salad: "I can't eat these leaves, nothing but leaves". I tried to convince him they were good for him but he wasn't having any of it. "I am from New York and used to big, red, juicy steaks," at which point he eagerly pulled out a colour brochure of his favourite steak restaurant and promptly showed us the picture of his favourite, juicy red steak! He looked at it with such longing.

After explaining that his wife had sadly died the year before and that he missed her dreadfully, he then added resignedly that his doctors in New York didn't feel he would make it to Christmas, He looked so broken. I asked him how long HE thought he would live, to which he replied after some thought: "two cruises! I have two cruises left in me". I didn't understand until later that each year he and his wife went on a cruise. Bearing this in mind, I interpreted his reply as meaning two years! Pretty good after being in hospital for only three days!

A few days later, I saw Al again on the ward looking very perky. He beckoned me over to sit with him in a cosy corner. I asked him how the cruises were going and his eyes lit up: *'I have four cruises in me now!'* Wow, four cruises after only six days treatment, I was thrilled. My wee cruiser had already extended his life by four years!

His good spirits didn't end there either. He started chatting me up!

> **A little advice**
>
> *Do not underestimate the power within you to change your attitude to your life and how you choose to live it!*

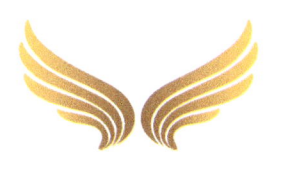

"I could find joy in the simplest of things and I never stopped being in awe of the beauty and majestic power of nature in all its glory".

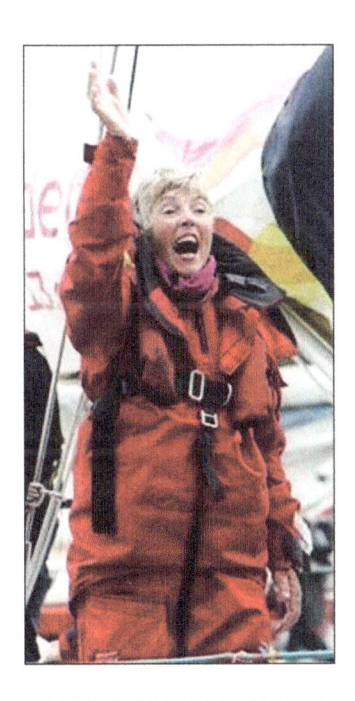

MICHELLE MCCANN

I grew up with Geraldine, my best friend and her sister Michelle in Derry, Northern Ireland. We spent lots of time together until I left to come to England to university when I was nineteen. I had not seen Michelle till last year, over forty years later. We met again at Café Soul where I was giving a talk to The Pink Ladies' Breast Cancer Support Group. I couldn't believe we were all sitting there together. Michelle looked radiant. All I could see was her amazing light.

Here Michelle shares her beautiful story of love and freedom through her husband's Dan's cancer:

I met my husband Dan when I was just thirteen years old. I didn't tell him that. I told him I was fifteen. I thought he would not be interested if he thought I was so young. He was fifteen. I thought he was a mature well-travelled man.

Our family took a house for a fortnight one August near the beach in Donegal. We had a lovely time there. The house did not have electricity and the heating and cooking was created by an old- fashioned turf-burning range. Dan was one of a group of locals that we made friends with. I fancied him at once but didn't tell anyone. My sister and I were sent to the shop one evening to get bread and I met up with Dan. We went for a walk to the beach and Dan held my hand. I got my first kiss at the beach and the loaf of bread got gently squashed!

He went to sea shortly after that because that was what he did, and I didn't see him again for a long time. He used to send me the occasional postcard from some foreign place like Ancona or Stavanger or Morocco. I never forgot him and, although I had other boyfriends, I hoped to meet him again some time.

In the summer when I was sixteen, I was at that same beach with my sister and her boyfriend and I met Dan again. It was partly due to good luck and partly because I walked up and down past his house in the hope that he would be at home and would see me. He was and he did. We went for a walk and we talked and talked and laughed. I felt very comfortable and easy with him and I found I still fancied him. That was really the beginning I suppose. He was still at sea at that time and we wrote to each other regularly. When he came home that Christmas he plucked up the courage to come up to my house and meet my parents. They liked him immediately, although they were not happy about me getting too serious at the age of sixteen. They had ambitions for me and wanted me to go to university after leaving school.

Dan and I fell head over heels in love with each other. We hated being separated and when he was at home we spent as much time as we could together. After a brief lonely time at college in England I eventually got a job in the civil service at home and we made plans to get married. We got married on 1st April when I was twenty-one and Dan was twenty-two. It was a happy day. Not the happiest, because the best was yet to come. Our son was born the following summer and life took on a new meaning for both of us. His brother, who arrived four years later, and sister, who was born another four years after that, gave us joy that we couldn't believe. We didn't know that parents could have such delight in their children like that. I can honestly say that our children gave us nothing but happiness all their lives.

Dan was still going to sea when we got married and both of us accepted that that would be the way of it. Seafaring families were common at the time in the community that we lived in. He worked very hard and studied hard and put himself through his Mates' ticket and then his Masters' ticket at the young age of twenty two. Fortunately shortly before our first son was born he got a job as Ship's Pilot following in the footsteps of his father, brother, uncle, grandparents and many generations before that. He stayed in that job then and was based at home which was wonderful.

When our children grew up a bit, I decided to go back to college and, with Dan's support and encouragement, I obtained first an HNC then a degree in computer studies. The subject I loved most, however, was mathematics and during the same period, through the Open University, I obtained my first class honours degree in mathematics. I could not have done that without the encouragement and support from Dan. While the children were small, I lectured part-time in our nearby higher education college and our university. I did a postgraduate certificate in education and began teaching mathematics on a full time basis in the grammar school that I had attended myself. I still work there and I love it.

Health was never a significant issue for us

Health was never a significant issue for us. The children had the usual childhood illnesses. Dan had trouble with his back periodically. When he was eighteen years old he first had problems with haemorrhoids, just as his father had experienced and it was something that occurred every now and then over the years. He had to get regular health check-ups due to his work and through these it was discovered that his blood pressure was quite high and that he had high cholesterol. That was surprising as he ate very well. Unlike me, Dan had no liking for sweet things, or fried food. He took medication for these conditions but it did not cause him any bother at all. And so our lives went on. We were very happy together and spent as much time with each other as possible. I still fancied him.

MICHELLE

Dan introduced me to sailing. We always had a boat of some sort and then when the children got older we bought a small yacht, upgrading to larger and more comfortable craft over the years. We spent as much time as we could on board the boat and every summer we spent our holidays sailing mainly about the Hebrides. The children sometimes came on trips but usually it was just the two of us. Dan was an excellent sailor and on board the boat he was the skipper without doubt. We had wonderful times on that boat.

One August we sailed to the Outer Hebrides and ended our trip on an island called Eriskey. It is a beautiful place that was one of our favourites. It is always hard to leave a place like that at the end of a holiday and begin to make our way south, but this time Dan seemed especially keen to go. His haemorrhoids were playing him up. He was tired and wanted to get home. That was unusual. He went back to work and continued as normal. However, a few weeks later he developed flu symptoms. There was a bad 'flu' going around that people were finding hard to shake off, so Dan was not concerned about his symptoms and got on with things as he usually did, taking the odd aspirin and lemon drink. His 'flu' symptoms came and went several times and he did not look well. He was able to continue working however and both of us assumed that it would soon pass. He was due for a routine medical and as part of that he was given liver function tests. The tests showed that there was something unusual going on but there seemed to be no cause for alarm and the doctor arranged for him to get a scan in a nearby hospital. Dan was not used to hospitals and felt it was alien territory to him. He fitted his scan in to a busy working day and didn't say too much about it at the time. Later he remarked that everyone seemed especially nice to him and that alarmed him. The doctor who did the scan spent a long time over it but eventually told Dan he would send the report on to Dan's own doctor. Dan felt that they wanted to say something more to him but he didn't really want to know at that time. He went on back to work.

The following weekend was extremely busy for him with regard to work and he had to go on several ships during the nights. He was not feeling very well. On the Sunday he got home some time during the night and lying in bed, he asked me to feel his tummy as he thought it seemed swollen. It was indeed and for the first time I felt a real fear deep down. He promised to go to the doctor the following day. He didn't. He went off to work and so did I. On my way home that evening I got a text message from him to get home straight away. I arrived home and Dan was waiting for me at the door. His face was white and he looked alarmed. He had received a call from his doctor to go to the surgery and to bring me with him. There was something unusual about the scan that he wanted to discuss with us.

The day our lives changed forever

The doctor had been our family doctor for a long time. He was the same age as Dan. He explained that the scan showed signs of cancer in several places on the liver but the primary site might be somewhere else. He was very kind and told us that he had already arranged for Dan to go to hospital the following morning. We heard his words but neither of us could take in what he was saying. We had so many questions but we had no voice. Dan was very ill. That night we lay together sleepless and close. We did not talk much except to repeat the positive things that had been said during the day. Inside I was screaming.

The following morning we set off for the hospital. On the way Dan stopped at the beach near our home that had been a part of his life since childhood. He got out of the car and stood alone looking out over the sand and the sea. When he came back his eyes were full. Dan, who hated hospitals got tested and tested. People were kind there though and as honest as they could be. We appreciated that, as it was a fear that he would not be told the truth about the extent of his illness. He was. As the tests went on the news got worse and worse. It seemed that the root of the problem was a small aggressive tumour in the bowel that had caused little or no symptoms on its own, apart from possibly the 'haemorrhoid-like' bleeding which we had ignored. The cancer however had spread from there to invade most of his liver. There were also signs of tumours in the lungs. Surgery was out of the question. And then there came a devastating statement.

Without treatment Dan would be lucky to have six months. With treatment "Who knows?" By the time this was said, however, we both really knew how serious his condition was, but it was difficult hearing it spoken out loud. Dan stayed in hospital for a few days and I stayed in with him. I slept in the hospital bed beside him because I didn't want to let him out of my sight. Our eldest son came home from abroad within 24 hours and the other two stayed with us for as long as they could. In their positive encouraging ways they allowed us to gradually come to terms with what was happening and reassure us that the treatment Dan received could extend his life considerably. It was essential to have the presence of our dear children there.

Dan came home from hospital soon after that and began treatment including chemotherapy as soon as possible. He did not lose his hair nor did he have any of the sickness associated with chemotherapy that people often experience. In fact he felt better than he had been feeling for a long time.

We had almost a year!

It was a good year. I mean, Dan was strong and well able to do things for himself. He maintained a good appetite for most of that time. He also maintained his wonderful sense of humour and we laughed a lot during that year. The children came to see us every day but it was not in sadness. We had our little granddaughter by then and she was a delight. Dan loved spending time with her. He read to her and told her stories. He sang her songs although he could not keep a tune. It was a joy to see them together. During the year also our eldest son had his first baby and they brought him half way across the world for Dan to meet. It seems bizarre, but that precious year counts among one of the happiest in my life. There was no time for sorrow. We didn't talk about the future and we didn't talk much about the past. We lived from moment to moment and that's what made it good.

From the beginning I felt that it was very important to keep the atmosphere around Dan calm and happy.

MICHELLE

The words I spoke were positive and hopeful, but at night when he was asleep I went down to the kitchen to look up the internet for more information about bowel cancer. I found some, but, in the early days especially, I was horrified by what I was reading. It was a lonely time. All my life since we were together, Dan was my best friend. He was my source of strength during the hard episodes of my life and now when I needed that strength of his I could not turn to him. I cried when I knew he could not see me and eventually I stopped looking for more information. Gradually I faced the fact that Dan was not going to recover. And then he began to comfort me. He knew what was happening to his body although he didn't look at the internet and he knew, as he always did, how I was really feeling. We clung to each other.

Apart from me and our children, Dan had many other people who loved him. He was the youngest, by far, of eight children. His eldest brother was twenty-three years older than him and they were all devastated by the news of his disease. The oncologist thought that the type of cancer Dan had was familial and suggested his brothers and sisters get tested but any tests on other members of his family proved negative. Early in his career at sea Dan had worked on board a ship that dumped nuclear waste and he sometimes wondered if that could have had anything to do with his cancer. The oncologist thought that was unlikely. She believed that the tumour had started with a polyp and quickly developed and spread.

On Sept 11th 2008, almost eleven months after he was first diagnosed, Dan died. It was only during the last couple of weeks that he felt tired and wanted to stay in bed. I stayed with him all the time. He wasn't frightened. He wasn't in pain and his passing was gentle. The nurse was in the house at the time and our daughter was there too. His funeral took place on a beautiful sunny autumn morning and it was a lovely celebration of his life.

I do feel grateful for that year we spent together

Then I had to learn to live without him. Apart from the grief they were feeling about losing their dear father, the children were also very worried about me and how I would cope. I needed to reassure them that I would be all right, so that's what I did. I was all right. I didn't go to pieces. I felt, and still do feel grateful for that year we spent together. I have very happy memories and I laugh often when I think of some of the things Dan got up to over the years. He loved me with all his heart, as I did him, and I will carry that with me forever.

I went back to work at the beginning of November, just over a year since the day I had left. I was glad to be back and I received genuine, warm support from my colleagues for which I was very grateful. I settled back into a regular routine of work and home. I try not to spend too much time analysing how I feel because there is nothing I can change and I try to see something good in every day that passes.

Reluctantly, after a few years, I put the boat up for sale. It was too much for me to handle on my own and it was sad to see it unused and neglected. It was a bad time to hope to sell a boat but I was very lucky because the original owner saw it up for sale and put in an offer. I was pleased to sell it to him, as I knew he would look after it well and enjoy it the way it was meant to be enjoyed. It was a very hard thing though to let it go, as it had been such a big part of our lives and we had such wonderful times on it.

I applied to sail the whole way around the world!

I missed sailing and I went on a brief sailing holiday in Scotland which I enjoyed. Then I read in my local newspaper a very interesting announcement. Derry City Council was going to sponsor one of the yachts that would be taking part in the Clipper Round the World Yacht Race in 2011/2012. This was an exciting venture for the city. I was familiar with the clipper race and had followed the previous race in 2009/2010. I looked it up online and saw that they were looking for crew. Slowly an idea began to develop in my mind that I would love to do a leg of the race. Dan and I had been planning to sail across the Atlantic when we retired from work. We were gradually preparing the boat for this and it was a dream that we were seriously intending to fulfil. I had given up on the idea that it would ever happen, then, with this announcement, the hope was reborn inside me.

I sent off for information which I received promptly, together with an application form. I studied the route and looked at the various legs, and I felt excited for the first time in a long time. I wanted to cross the Atlantic, but I also wanted to sail the Southern Ocean. I wanted to sail the first leg out of Europe and across the Equator. I wanted to transit the Panama Canal. Ah, it was all just too much. I couldn't decide which leg I wanted to do the most. Well, why not all of it? So that's what I did. I applied to go the whole way around the world. The Clipper Ventures' organisers came to Derry to promote the race and I had an interview. It was in a hotel in Derry and as I was being interviewed, a song was being played over the PA system. It was a Van Morrison song that meant a lot to Dan and I, and I smiled to myself. It was meant to be? I was accepted! I couldn't believe it. I hadn't told anyone that I was applying in case I was turned down or changed my mind. After hearing that I was accepted, I laughed all the way home in the car. My family was dumbstruck.

I was granted a year's career break from school and so began my preparations for the year long trip. I did all the required training in England said my goodbyes to family and friends and then, on 31st July 2011, we departed Southampton for our epic voyage on board the Clipper 68 yacht 'Derry Londonderry'.

It was everything I hoped it would be and more

The trip lasted for a full year and on 22nd July 2012 we sailed triumphantly back into Southampton, completing our circumnavigation of over 43,000 miles. I had a wonderful trip. It was everything I hoped it would be and more. We had some glorious weather at times and we saw beautiful sunsets, sunrises, magical night skies and amazing wildlife. On one occasion a whale emerged from the sea just a few metres from the boat. Another time we almost collided with one! We saw many dolphins, sea turtles, flying fish, albatrosses and other wildlife that I had previously only ever read about.

MICHELLE

Oh, we had some awful weather too, with winds reaching up to 50 knots in the Southern Ocean. The Pacific crossing was tough. We had one storm after another and that went on for more than four weeks with winds up to force 11. It was a similar story during our final Atlantic crossing from Nova Scotia to Derry, when again we had to deal with force 11. That was very hard, but we made it and there was a terrific sense of achievement when we arrived safely at each port, regardless of our position in the race.

I had to work very hard most of the time, harder than I've ever worked in my life, lifting sails, grinding winches, cleaning bilges etc. as well as helming and trimming the sails. Conditions were very wet, cold and uncomfortable at times. I had a few scary moments, but only one or two where I was really frightened and that's not bad over the course of a year. Some of the worst weather gave the most exciting sailing and I loved it.

On 30th June 2012 after battling with the Atlantic Ocean and hurricane 'Chris' for almost three weeks we were approaching the west coast of Ireland. Imagine my delight, when I realised that the dark patch I could see on the horizon through the dark grey rain was actually a mountain range in County Sligo. After having been away for so long I felt very emotional at the prospect of coming home.

We arrived at the mouth of the river Foyle the following morning and sailed up to the finish line. This is where I live and there it was. There was the beach that meant so much to me. A bonfire was lit on the hill to welcome us. We were greeted by my son who came out to meet us in his own boat and as the morning went on many other local boats joined us. As we made our way up the Lough, it seemed that we were escorted by every vessel in the area that could float. The pilot boat came out and the pilot came on board. He was a colleague of Dan's and a life-long family friend. All the way up the river there were people waving and cheering. I saw banners with "Welcome Home Michelle" written on them. Our boat had sailed under many famous bridges around the world, but to my eyes, the Foyle Bridge was the most beautiful sight as we sailed under it towards Derry, the city where I was born, grew up and worked. On the quayside there were thousands of people out cheering and waving. What a welcome we received! I was very proud of my homeland and I will never forget that day.

I learned a lot during that year and discovered courage and strengths I never knew I had. I learned that *I could find joy in the simplest of things and I never stopped being in awe of the beauty and majestic power of nature in all its glory.* Dan was ever present. I felt him with me and that made me smile. When we crossed the Atlantic Ocean for the first time I felt a terrific sense of achievement and satisfaction that our ambition had been fulfilled.

I found the way forward
I think somehow during that year I found the way forward. I had a lot of time to think during long quiet

watches and I became aware of just how lucky I have been in life. I have a loving family and dear friends. I have good health and no real money worries. I have been blessed with an optimistic happy nature, but best of all, I have lived most of my life loving and being loved by a wonderful man. I have laughed a lot and I treasure many memories of the fun we had. I believe it is an honour to Dan to remember him with joy and not sadness and to look forward to the future with enthusiasm and hope. The world is beautiful and I want to experience more of it while I can.

A little advice

Nothing in life can prepare you for dealing with this, so be patient and do what is right for you and your partner. Although it is tempting to talk about the past and happy occasions, I found that this made Dan uncomfortable and a little sad, as did talking too much about the future. Stay in the present moment and enjoy every minute of your time together. Now is the time for 100% unconditional love. Don't be afraid.

"God, I thank you for this pain"

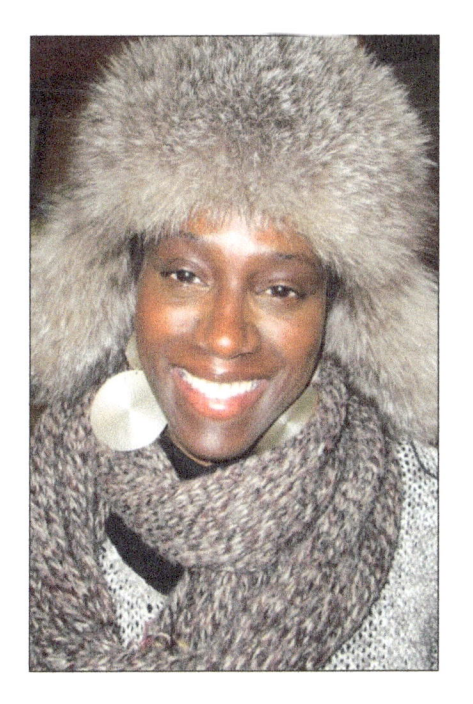

JAY DAVIDSON

I met Jay at the 'Living Wholehearted' retreat for cancer patients and their partners/carers at The Global Retreat Centre in Nuneham Courtney in Oxfordshire in 2012. Jay was part of a panel of individuals including myself who were sharing their healing experiences through cancer. What struck me about Jay was her unshakeable focus on healing herself through her nightmare. She exuded a brilliant light within.

Here is Jay's impassioned learning and healing through cancer:

Hi I'm Jay and I live in London. I was diagnosed with Multiple Myeloma, a rare form of leukaemia, both the bone marrow and blood. I was diagnosed on Christmas Eve 2010 after months of aches and pains in my middle and lower back. At the time of diagnosis I worked in the action-packed, highly social London media industry; a life full of action, where I worked hard and played harder with my fabulous friends. It's not a life I could ever have complained about.

What am I?
Since leaving university, I sailed through various different glamorous jobs including working with super stars and pop stars and big record labels. Later I moved into the world of radio and TV. That was my life really. I enjoyed life and socialised a lot. When I reached my 30th, I started reading spiritual books and little did I know what a massive part my understanding of what I read would play in my life. I read books like 'Conversations with God' and 'The Way of the Peaceful Warrior'. Books like these woke me from a slumber. My new perception of God wasn't the one I learned about in Sunday school. That God didn't make sense to me – that God was in my mind, a contradiction of an often angry, yet loving parent – punishing and rewarding and easy to offend. I always had an awareness of 'myself' and I do remember, at nine years of age, asking about who am I and looking at my hand, wondering: What am I? That feeling of looking at my hand but knowing I am not my hand intrigued me. As for the spiritual books – I would read and be inspired by them, then put them down and then continue living life. I was always into taking care of my body physically and was an athlete

throughout school and college. Later I discovered yoga and absolutely loved it, but it wasn't until one of my best friends introduced me to Bikram Yoga that I began to practise several times a week. I loved how it made me feel and, just like the spiritual books, helped to prepare me for the future. Up to the point of diagnosis, my understanding of the books was from an intellectual level. I agreed with it, what I was reading, but I wasn't really living it, and deep down I knew it. I was in a relationship with a man that wasn't really right. It was somebody that I really loved and still love now. But he could see my inconsistencies: between who I was being, between the books on my shelf and the person that I was. We decided to call it a day that year, which plunged me into all sorts of emotional turmoil, of not 'being good enough'. I was devastated.

God, I thank you for this pain!

About three months later, my body was just not feeling right. Nevertheless, I started with Bikram Yoga 30 Day Challenge, practising it every day for a month, which is quite heavy going. A week into the challenge though, I had to stop because my back was in agony. I thought I had injured myself in the yoga studio. I went to see the doctor over several weeks and was given painkillers and sent on my way. But they didn't work. I went back: more painkillers. I was on super-high doses which only succeeded in temporarily masking the pain, whilst making me constipated. I started to ask: "What IS this pain?" I could no longer practise yoga because it hurt my back so much. My left buttock was really tight which became more severe when I sat down which wasn't right after two months coming and going to doctors and having sport's massage. Nothing worked. I went to an acupuncturist and explained the pain and even identified the muscle that was causing it. The acupuncture worked and took the pain away – I was so relieved! It was the first time in months that I was pain-free. But, within an hour of getting home, the pain returned and it was the most unbearable pain I had experienced so far. I remember leaning against the heat of the radiator and saying out loud and quietly inwardly at the same time: "*God, I thank you for this pain! I THANK YOU FOR THIS PAIN! I don't know what this pain is, or why it's there, but I surrender it to you*". I trusted that something good had to come from this.

Back on the painkillers and it was not long after that when I spoke to a friend who is also a personal trainer. She asked if I had seen a physiotherapist. She told me of the amount of times she and her colleagues have come across clients who complain of aches and pains, yet never go to a physiotherapist about it. She suggested one who was the husband of a work colleague and mutual friend. So, for the cost of £60, I could see him. It never crossed my mind to go to my GP to get referred. I had spent half an hour talking to him and half an hour with him examining me.

On the back of this hour, he wrote a letter to my GP and said: "From what I have seen, you need an MRI scan".

Two days later, I was back in my doctor's office. He gave me yet another prescription for a different type of pain reliever but, to his credit, he decided to get me the scan as the physio had suggested. As I went to go out the door, something greater than me turned me around and I asked: "Actually, as you are about to fax off the referral for the MRI, could you write my telephone number on the form?" It was the week before Christmas – the post would've taken ages. Three days later, I had a phone call offering me an appointment for the end of January. I knew I couldn't wait till then, with the pain I was in. I just need to get it sorted. Remarkably, and like an angel, the voice down the phone asked: "Can you do tomorrow?" It turned out that there was an appointment available in Harley Street. I was so weak that I had to take a taxi there. I did the scan and felt so rough that I couldn't even leave after. I laid down in this side room for a while. The nurses refused to let me go on public transport and put me in a cab and sent me on my way.

I went back to work and my boss took one look at me and said: 'You, young lady are getting into a cab straight out of here". She sent me to my grandma's house. On the way there, I stopped off with a prescription my doctor had given me, to pick up the painkillers. I remember opening up the packet and one of the side effects was suicidal thoughts. I never took one. Forget that! Then ..., well! Then I had to wait. I never forgot the words from the doctor's office on receiving my scan results. "You need you to go to Casualty right now and we need to admit you straight away. We have seen something on the scan which is of concern to us. There is a soft tissue mass on your spine and it is pressing on your spinal cord. That's what's been causing the pain."

No Way!

I jumped into the cab with my Gran and called two of my friends on the way: one wasn't in but Deborah answered. She dropped whatever she was doing and met me at the hospital. I was in there for a few hours. Another friend – more like big sis, Valerie, turned up to support. The docs had their suspicions: "Whatever it is, it's nasty" and said they would have to admit me that evening. The following day would be spent going through a series of doing different biopsies, scans, blood tests and X-Rays, so they wanted to start early first thing in the morning – Christmas Eve. It was so freaking surreal like: "How can this be really happening?!" The next day Deborah returned to the hospital. By now I was on a ward. Bless her heart: she sat in my room, reading magazines as I was being wheeled in and out for different procedures, being prodded and poked and pricked by needles again and again. Finally, at about 6.30pm, they came to inform me of the diagnosis: "So we are sorry to have to tell you we have found cancer". I was squeezing Deb's hand, but said: "No way!" That was the first thing that came out of my mouth. They said: "And that's the attitude you need to have!" Nevertheless, it was incredibly tough news as we lost a beautiful friend, Brian Daley, aka DJ Swing, not 5 years before. I turned to Debs: "I'm so sorry to put you through all of this again." My friends were incredible and you will hear me talk about my friends like they were just my angels. They stepped up to the plate and goodness knows what they must have been going through. I get a little sense of that now. My friends shielded me from how they really felt seeing me so ill. The next day was Christmas Day, the day after so much had happened. I had a lot of visitors, despite the awful snowy conditions outside. The mother of a friend sent in Christmas dinner for me and we ate lamb, turkey with rice and peas and all the trimmings. I ate all of it and what I couldn't eat I kept in the fridge. I had a stereo for music. It was all very jolly in my room. This entire ward had individual rooms and on the door of my room it said: "You are entering a healing zone!" I had pictures and lots of cards that came and I put up pictures of people I loved and who were really giving, amazing and supportive. I remember more of that than I do of the treatment. The doctors were coming in and out, explaining that I would need to start chemo really soon. I would listen to music, read, dance and pray and thought about nothing but my recovery. They also told me that any treatment was likely to make me infertile. So I had to go through that realisation and the decision being taken out of my hands. I was very pragmatic about it and it didn't take me too long to agree, as freezing eggs would have taken time for something which isn't even a guaranteed procedure – time that I wouldn't get back. I had a word with myself: "Well, you are here. I am what is important here, not a child that doesn't actually exist". So I chose there and then that I'd give myself the best possible chance for survival. If the time comes when I want to have a child, I am sure that there will be a child for me to love; it doesn't necessarily have to be one to whom I physically give birth.

So I started the treatment. When the nurses came in to give me chemotherapy intravenously, it always came in a black bag because it needed to be protected from the light. I ordered heart-shaped 'post-it' notes and I stuck a couple on the black chemo bag and around my room. I stayed in hospital for three weeks and I really wanted to know how this had happened. I was a healthy eater, I practised yoga, gave up cigarettes seven years prior to this. How could I be this ill? One of my friends suggested talking to her psychic healer, Molly. She'd really helped her in the past and was also working with another one of my other friends too. So I called to speak to this woman. She asked why I thought I was unwell but I didn't know. She said: "What I am getting here, Jay, is that your life needs to take a different path. You are not living the life you should be living". That made sense to me and she said: "Ok, but why did it have to be so drastic! I know people need to wake up, but this is a very drastic way to wake someone up isn't it?" And, almost immediately, I knew the answer. I said it as she said it: "She wouldn't have listened otherwise." Ah, that's so true.

After a week of being there, I was seen by a lovely orthopaedic surgeon who examined my spine. He was concerned to discover I had a fracture and my spine appeared weakened and vulnerable. He decided that I was to be put in a back brace which would extend from my neck to my hips to keep my spine stable until he could operate. Because it was in the middle of the holidays, the soonest I could get a brace fitted was a week later in the New Year, so, until that time, he put me on bed rest, without being able to sit up more than 45 degrees. So it was bed pan and bed washes. It's amazing what your mind does when you are told you cannot leave your bed. In my dreams, I was out of the ward: my body left and I was off. I had a dream: I was in the fridge down the corridor from my room and I think I remember asking this guy to pass me the fork and him saying I would get him into trouble as he should not be out here. I knew I should be lying down. I woke up. This was hilarious. There was another dream where I had jumped back into my body and woke up with a startling jump and I was like: "Well, ok, that was a trip!' Eventually, after three weeks hospitalisation, they let me out. Feeling the fresh air on my face was terrific. I hadn't felt fresh air for three or four weeks' – outside breeze and outside air. I felt weak and fragile. I felt smaller. I felt unwell.

All my protectiveness/defensiveness evaporated

2011 was a very long year of treatment. Results would go up and then go down. My parents flew over to be with me and I wouldn't let them in. I was very gung-ho about this. Bless my parents! I would leave them with no room to manoeuvre, repeatedly telling them that I was fine. They felt useless because I wouldn't let them in. In some weird way, I thought I was protecting them. Later, I understood that you can never stop a parent from worrying about their child. Meanwhile, the treatment continued. The results were coming back with partial success – one step forward, two steps backward. All the docs were getting very concerned. The cancer had attacked my spine which was so fragile that I had 2 fractures and had to wear a back brace to protect it.

I was even banned from practising yoga. That was a pretty big deal for a yoga fan like me.

It was a funny existence. I was having regular sessions with Molly, yet I felt cloudy and muddy. The docs took care of the medical side, whilst I did all manner of alternative treatments. It gave me some sense of control and helped keep my mind in order. One day, Molly called to say she was at a session for Theta healers in Kensington and that they need people to train as part of a training day. They were experienced Theta healers but they still needed people to work on. I don't know how she found out about it but she said that they were doing one the next day and felt that I should come along and get some healing. Basically, I grabbed any healing sessions that came my way; I lapped it up. So off I went to the Theta Healing group. Myself and three or four others sat in this spacious room and around the walls were healers. The leader said: "Right, choose whomever you feel drawn to and speak to that person". I was immediately drawn to this particular woman with pink and purple hair; an amazing, lovely woman whom I still know to this day and, it turns out, happened to be a breast cancer survivor. We started speaking and she wanted to know more about my family. As soon as I started talking about them, I burst into tears. Immediately, the senior lady who was running the whole workshop came over and said: "Oh, something is going on here!" We got to the root, that I hadn't mourned my family emigrating when I was nineteen and it had stayed in my psyche. I just got on with life but it affected me in more ways than I could have imagined. I didn't deal with it. She asked how it was, when they came to visit and I explained that I was protecting them. She said that you do not need to protect your parents. They are your parents and nothing you do can stop them worrying about you, so you might as well let them get involved. As your parents, it's their job and there's nothing you can do to stop it all changing. But I was also very protective of my mum, in particular. We had worked on some very deep issues concerning a member of the family who was not being very nice to her when I was a child. "Well you are going to need to talk to your mum about it soon" but I explained that I didn't think I could do this. That evening I called home and my dad answered the phone. I didn't expect her to be home from work yet and I was surprised when he told me she was. She asked me where I was today and we were on the phone for an hour. I told her about my healing session and, to my surprise, she said it made total sense to her. We definitely had a clearing that evening, my mum and I. All my protectiveness/defensiveness had evaporated and my mum had her girl back.

"What can I learn from you, tree?

From the early stages of my treatment, I understood that my healing was mind, body and spirit. The doctors were doing their body part and I was doing the mind and spirit part – finding places like Brahma Kumaris, Molly the psychic healer, people like Topaz, my healer, books by Wayne Dyer, Louise Hay and Michael Beckwith – but not so much reading them but feeling and truly understanding the principles. All these books had a common thread about them. Our bodies are amazing machines, yet thought affects our bodies at a cellular level. What we eat, we become. And thoughts are very powerful. I was getting this recurring theme from more than one source and I absorbed the stuff that resonated with me most. I also prayed a lot. One of my cousins is very powerful in prayer and she would come and pray over me. Her prayer was so powerful that she would start speaking in tongues and all sorts. This was the energy I was around and any friends who were either afraid of what I was going through or just unable to handle it, disappeared and were replaced by friends that were so loving and supportive that I had a beautiful bubble of care around me. I lost an incredible amount of weight, going down to six stone; healthy weight being just over or just under 9 stone. At that point, I had to say goodbye to my hair. I had very long hair and, at first, the realization hit hard; but even then I dug deep as a way of getting my head around it. I knew if I am crying this much for my hair, it needed to go because it's an attachment. Let it go. It's just hair; it will grow back. But we identify with all this external stuff don't we? By then I was incredibly weak. One month later, after shaving my head, I went to The Global Retreat Centre. By now, walking was a real effort for me. It was in the grounds of this beautiful, stately home in the middle of the Oxfordshire countryside that I met Mr. Redwood – a giant redwood tree. I had a moment on my own with him and I looked up at his massive trunk. I thought to myself, I am going to come back and see you one day Mr Redwood. I was annoyed as I hadn't taken my i-phone with me to take a picture. I don't know why, but I needed to have a picture of this tree. "What can I learn from you, tree?"

JAY

He said "Strength. There is just as much strength in you as there is in me".

About two weeks later, I had to go back into hospital as I had another fracture in my spine; this time in my lower spine. So, whilst I was there, I got a phone call from my doctor who asked me: "What are you doing there Jay!?" I explained that I had another fracture in my spine and she said: "I need you to get to this other hospital tomorrow because you need to have radiotherapy". So I literally left one hospital, came home, changed my clothes and went to another hospital to have radiotherapy. It was crazy. I did five days of that and it was tough. They targeted my stomach area which played havoc with my digestion. I just couldn't eat anything. Everything tasted the same: wet cardboard, dry cardboard, warm, and cool cardboard. I remember, on the 5th day, the hospital called me up and said: "Well, we will admit you for your stem cell transplant on Monday". "Can't I have a break, I am exhausted?" She said: "No I am sorry, you will have to come in; we can't wait with you anymore". I didn't realise what was going on behind the scenes: they were incredibly concerned for me. "We need you to come in on Monday."

The night before I went in, I got to the stage where I couldn't bathe myself. I could clothe myself but not bathe. My grandmother, who was by then in her eighties, would sit me in a small bath and sitting on her plastic stool, she would bathe me and dry me off. My grandma is a former nurse and my hero – a giant of a woman – even though she's barely 5 feet tall. The night before

I went into hospital for the last time, I was bald and naked. Standing in my bedroom I asked myself: "I am doing all the positive things: eating well, meditating etc., why is this cancer still here?" And I was really asking: What am I missing here? I don't get it. There is something I was definitely not getting." I began reading a book by Marianne Williamson's bestseller, 'A Return to Love'. Something had drawn me to pick it up. It is a beautiful book and I would encourage everyone to read it if they can. Pretty much everyone will find something relevant to them and there was a lot in this book relevant to me, including this gem of wisdom:

Our Deepest Fear

Our deepest fear is not that we are inadequate.
Our deepest fear is that we are powerful beyond measure.
It is our light, not our darkness
That most frightens us.

We ask ourselves
Who am I to be brilliant, gorgeous, talented, fabulous?
Actually, who are you *not* to be?
You are a child of God.

Your playing small
Does not serve the world.
There's nothing enlightened about shrinking
So that other people won't feel insecure around you.

We are all meant to shine,
As children do.

JAY

We were born to make manifest
The glory of God that is within us.

It's not just in some of us;
It's in everyone.

And as we let our own light shine, we unconsciously give other people permission to do the same. As we're liberated from our own fear our presence automatically liberates others.

It's a beautiful moment in the book, so special that Nelson Mandela read this segment during his inaugural speech of his presidency. In another chapter, there was one particular line that jumped off the page: "God's plan works, yours doesn't". I had what Oprah calls an 'Aha!' moment! I need to refer to that line often. I realised that the reason I wasn't getting better was because I was trying to solve the problem and it wasn't my problem to solve. I needed to hand this one over. I started to pray: "I have no business trying to fix this. I am handing this over to you, not necessarily to do the healing, but if I trust in you there is no healing to be had". In other words, once you trust and know who you are and of your Divine connection, that, in itself, is the healing. Once you know yourself and trust in God, all the rest is an illusion. It's kind of like we make stuff up: "It's not from God, it's not divine: we don't deserve love, we don't deserve health, we don't deserve abundance etc. Whatever it is that separates us from what we really are, I surrender this situation over to you. I trust you with every beat of my heart. I hand this over to you." As I said it I was in tears.

> **A little advice**
>
> *I had my last session of chemo that month – less than 6 months later I was told I was clear, and I've been clear ever since. I never once owned it. I never once referred to being ill as 'my' cancer. I told the doctors to refer to it as such too. It took them some time, but they got it. It may have been there but it wasn't there to stay ...*

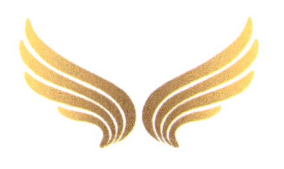

'If cancer is a messenger, it has an urgent message; if I can interpret that, I stand some chance of putting it right'.

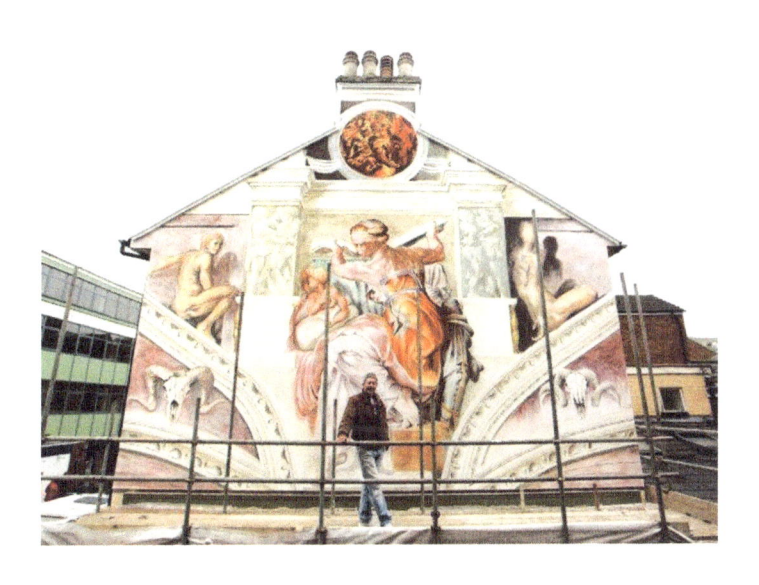

IAIN CARSTAIRS

IAIN and I met via The Issels Clinic in Mexico where Iain went for treatment for inoperable cancer last year. In light of his devastating diagnosis, Iain chooses to become involved in the healing process, learn everything possible about cancer, contributed by others all over the world, and try to overcome it on his own. His positivity, staggering research, belief and determination to heal himself whilst being a single parent of two children and, having overcome eye cancer nine years earlier, dumbfounded me. Being an artist, he was painting a fresco on one side of his own home in Bedford, completing eight months of work in June this year whilst actively committing himself to his own daily pro-active cancer treatment regime. At the same time he attended hospital to discover his tumour had reduced by his own actions!

Here Iain shares his resourceful, healing story with you:

It's never a good sign when after an endless battery of tests, a surgeon advises you to prepare for a lengthy course of drastic treatments, saying it will be "at least a year" before you feel you have survived the treatments alone! My old friend cancer seems to have made a meandering return; our introduction was literally a poke in the eye with something sharp. This time, it's more obvious and a lot bigger. 2002's Choroidal Melanoma was barely 2mm but made its presence inescapably obvious by its lifting of the retina. The advice that I had a 70% chance of surviving five years, razed my confidence to the ground, but proved wildly pessimistic. After five biopsies, an internal exam with a metal snake, blood tests, x-ray, ultrasound, MRI and the most impressive of the lot, a PET scan after which I was radioactive for a week, I have the final opinion: squamous cell carcinoma; a 1.5cm tumour at the base of the tongue on one side, and a secondary tumour in the adjacent submandibular lymph which PET technicians say show a 3cm area of "highly suspicious glucose uptake". Both John Diamond and Michael Douglas had the same kind of problem, with very different results.

Two Pleasing Choices!

So here was one choice: be out of action for a year, lose all the glands in my face and neck, have the back of my tongue burned away, and endure multiple doses of chemo – and after that have a forty per cent chance of a five year survival for someone in my stage 3 state. What about work? I can't be off the grid for even a few weeks. "It's unlikely you'll be able to work during that year," was the reply. When a surgeon says "unlikely" what he really wants to say is: "forget about it! Completely! Are you nuts?!" just as: "there may be some discomfort" translates to: "you'll enter a world of pain". I later mentioned that I'd wanted to consult with friends and family who underwent chemo, to get their opinion. "And..?" he ventured. "They're all dead."

But here's the other choice: an opportunity to become involved in the healing process, rather than be just a bystander; learn everything possible about cancer, from the vast amount of research and experience contributed by others all over the world, and try to overcome it on my own. The surgeon did his professional best to hide his despair, but reminded me this kind of cancer can spread to the cheek, and eventually to the brain. After three months he could not guarantee any worthwhile treatment. But sometimes life doesn't give you two pleasing choices, perhaps because, if it did, you could spend a lifetime dithering. So some decisions are surprisingly easy, and once made, a weight was lifted off me, and I felt free.

After the initial shock, I realised there were a few things actually in my favour. For one thing, my life is flexible enough that I can do any amount of research and re-work my diet in any direction without affecting my children or the quality of my technical output. The other advantage is an intense curiosity about molecules, how they work, and, not least, I have a faith that everything must have a reason. We live in a law-bound universe, from the molecules to the stars. The machinery of our body, above all else, is a process of order, not chaos. I do not believe in Darwin's idea that at the base of us is a hollow nothing. At the base of us is order, so concentrated and so intense that it forms an endless field of study. *If cancer is a messenger, it has an urgent message. If I can interpret that, I stand some chance of putting it right.* Cancer got a foothold at a certain time, which must say something about conditions at the cellular level, and I want to know what they are. I don't believe Nature intended mankind to develop scurvy or cancer. The two can be equated because, though symptoms are extreme, they are indeed symptoms, and the causes must be relatively simple – because life doesn't particularly favour the polymath. In some societies, cancer is virtually unknown. Japanese women have a very low incidence of breast cancer, but when they move to America, they develop tumours at the standard Western rate. Their genetics remain unaltered, presumably, which only leaves environment, including stresses, and diet. Armed with that faith, I begin my investigation. We'll learn how to approach it, or how not to and, in the process, uncover something which is bound to be extremely interesting.

What They Don't Tell You About Cancer

My diet for at least the year prior to turning to the doctors to see what this annoying lump was in my neck, consisted of endless espressos, white wine, pasta, stress and overwork. And in two final, freezing months, I had been working flat out on the construction of the first outdoor fresco in the UK, for which I was supremely unqualified: 15 hour days in a panic-ridden state of tension trying to finish applying pigments before the plaster dried, knowing that any variation in line or tone meant hacking the day's work off and starting again, as well as doing the school runs and maintaining the flow of emails and crises at work. And, as bad situations always get worse, it was over a coffee shop – the owner helpfully offering unlimited amounts in the hope of getting it done quicker.

I immediately jettisoned coffee, alcohol, and sugar (as far as it could be detected) and put together a plan of action to boost my immune system, using beta glucans, vitamins and minerals, as well as the body's pH (alkalinity and acidity balance), to try and make my body an unsuitable place for tumours so the existing pair would find it hard to metastasize. If it was unlikely to get worse, I could attack it with anything research or other people had found useful. I had never thought of food as medicine before, but that's exactly what it is.

I am not a gambling man

I want to say a big thanks to everyone who wrote or offered their support and good wishes. It was much appreciated because the worst thing about the word 'cancer' is the reaction it can cause in those who project a lifetime of media tragedies onto 'you'. It's especially hard for an impressionable person to avoid buying into what other people think. A well-meaning neighbour who lost his wife last year to the ravages of chemo, shook his head sadly and sympathised, "once it gets to the lymph, that's really it." That's why I stay away from hospitals: like a court of justice, their authority is easily mocked from afar. But once in either dock, when your life and times count for nothing, you start to wonder – can *all* these earnest people really be wrong? – and it dawns that a single shake of the head could change life for good.

So last Friday, with some trepidation, I met with my surgeon, a man to whom I already owe a great debt for his patience and experience. A month previously he couldn't guarantee anything useful could be done by the end of May, if I insisted on going my own way. We met as planned, despite his surgery running 40 minutes late. "How was I? Still averse to the radiation, radical neck dissection and chemo?" " I'm afraid so." "You have loads of patients," I ventured, "I can be, you know, the control group." He seemed appalled; "I don't want you to be the control group!" was said with genuine concern. Were they always doomed? I hadn't realised. "How about I take another biopsy while you're here?" "No, but thanks anyway!" "Mr Carstairs, as these things progress, in future I can't promise we can offer a cure, though we would of course still offer to treat you," he said, hoping the difference between two words might somehow sink in. "As you know, I can't force you to accept these procedures against your will," he conceded wistfully. He checked the neck, glands, etc, and we agreed the secondary tumour had not increased in size. "I'll check the primary tumour," and donning a plastic glove he made an internal exam of the very base of my tongue, seeming to use quite a bit of pressure. "Well?" "I can't seem to locate it..." We agreed to meet at the end of August, three months away. That's actually the minimum space between appointments for all the protocols I am on which treat the patient gradually, rather than the tumour suddenly, and are likely to have a noticeable effect on a tumour ensconced within the lymph node, now the size of a golf ball. As it turns out, my 40 minutes of elevated heart rate in reception were well spent: slowly chewing through an entire bag of almonds, ensuring the alkalinity of my saliva skyrocketed off the scale for a while. Plato said "We are twice armed, who fight with faith". Despite how it seems, I'm not a gambling man!

I packed a bag and headed off

According to its guidebook, the original Santa Barbara Mission in Southern California, established on the Feast of St Barbara, December 4, 1786 was the tenth of twenty one such Californian Missions founded by the Spanish Franciscans, and built by skilled Mexican labour. Be that as it may, my own Santa Barbara mission two hundred and twenty six years later was to deal with my nasty case of Squamous Cell Carcinoma that, if left untreated, I was reliably informed, would remove from me all the cares of this world in around 18 months' time. The plan of two separate specialists was to subject me to major surgery, chemo and radiation, which would take *about a year,* with a slim chance of this extending my planetary residence by six months. Mentioned obliquely was the chance of severing in the process vital nerves currently holding up the corners of my mouth and controlling my shoulders, along with a promise of losing every gland from cheekbones to shoulders on both sides – lymph, salivary alike – for good. Your maths being as good as mine, you'll understand why, instead of ingesting poison and thrusting my head into a radioactive guillotine, I packed a bag and headed off to a dedicated immunological clinic in Southern California.

Most people will never have heard of Josef Issels (1907 – 1998), the father of modern immunological medicine, but that's not for any want of effort on his part. His work was extraordinarily successful because he understood that the first appearance of a cancerous tumour, no matter how small, was already the final act in a chronic breakdown of the patient's immunological defences – defences which might have quietly eliminated cancer for decades beforehand. Josef Issels' treatments used every possible method to boost the immune system, often in tandem with surgery, and had remarkable results. Issels was a determined man, perfectly prepared to risk his own career to help patients. He flouted Nazi law in the late 1930's by treating German and Jewish patients alike, a humanitarian attitude the authorities punished by sending him to the Eastern Front as a medic. He was captured by the Russians and was lucky to survive four years in one of Stalin's slave labour camps. Afterwards Issels returned to start a medical practice in Germany, and in 1951 founded the first European hospital for "incurable" cancer patients. Issels later wrote an excellent book called 'Cancer: A Second Opinion' which is so dense with information I'm reading it a second time, and which I highly recommend to anyone with cancer, or who knows someone with cancer, or even those to whom cancer is only a shadow lurking in the corners of the mind, prodded back to life by regular media reports.

Rather than me list the complicated treatments I underwent over a period of weeks, you might prefer to hear that the staff and knowledge at the Issels Medical Centre are the best you're likely to find anywhere. This place is where hard-headed realism meets outside-the-box thinking, and where complex DNA and blood work and of course more than 60 years of immunological know-how meet the patient in a supportive and healthy environment. Whilst spending a month here in Santa Barbara, I allowed myself to think beyond the next year and imagine seeing my children grow, making new art, and perhaps seeing the world find solutions to the thorny problems which plague it.

Don't go back and do the same thing- it's not working!

In California the son of the famed Joseph Issels, Christian Issels stared at me over his desk: "when you go back, don't go back and do the same thing- it's not working." So now I give myself more time for technical projects rather than trying to impress with speed of delivery. People aren't impressed with speed unless they understand the difficulty of the job, and they can't be expected to. The faster you deliver, the less people think it is worth. There's no hurry – maybe despite what the doctors say, you've got time.

It's been twelve months since I was diagnosed with cancer and, judging by the reactions of the doctors, I seem to have already beaten the odds, which leads me to believe I will in all likelihood continue to do so. If anyone thinks I flouted medical recommendations out of recklessness, they'd be mistaken. I refused chemo, radical neck dissection and radiation only because none of them work worth a damn. Maybe people turn to chemo because they don't want to change anything in their life, or don't understand the problem, or because of wishful thinking that if someone else tackles it they'll succeed; despite the chaos having welled up for years from within, they expect a cure to come from a flame-thrower outside.

Let's look at what a person can do for themselves. If conditions in my body had created the tumours, only reversing them could stop the spread, if not dismantle them. You can drastically reduce the toxins you're absorbing every day. Changing the habits of a lifetime to turn the body around is bound to take time. But there are loads of other things a person can do.

1. So the first thing I did was get rid of all sugars, processed food, coffee and alcohol in my diet. This meant, respectively, that the tumours were no longer getting the glucose energy they needed to grow, I was no longer ingesting saturated fat molecules which were slowly suffocating my cells, and I was no longer reducing my (intracellular) pH levels.
2. I replaced these with juiced vegetables, the Budwig diet, and as much organic produce as I could get. These steps in turn provided fresh enzymes and raised my pH and started to reinvigorate my cell respiration with healthy unsaturated fat molecules. I no longer had to worry about genetically polluted food loaded with toxins and pesticides.
3. Aftershave or perfume without 'fragance' – Any aftershave or perfume with "fragrance" on the label already has at least 400 chemicals in it which the skin and glands will absorb.
4. Mineral Water – Drinking mineral water instead of tap water means you're no longer accumulating fluoride which is not naturally occurring fluoride

but toxic waste called either sodium fluoride or hydrofluosilicic acid as described as an "unstable, poisonous corrosive", in your own body.

5. Natural Shampoo – Changing shampoo from a tar-based (carcinogenic) product to a natural one, and using a fluoride-free toothpaste, further reduces the load on the struggling immune system.

6. Even dental floss comes with a coating of teflon and petroleum –natural silk floss lasts longer. Stop using vaseline on your lips, as it's only a short hop away from gasoline. How do you think they came up with the name?

7. Enzymes like bromelain, papain, trypsin and chymotrypsin can be obtained in capsule form, and they gradually chip away at the tough protection around tumours. Bromelain comes from pineapples, concentrated in the core, and remains potent even as the fruit rots. Papain comes from the papaya fruit and works best at higher temperatures, so is perfect for feeding to the body in papaya tea.

8. Melons – In melons there is another enzyme the body makes less of as you grow older: superoxide dismutase.

9. Sunshine – The other thing I do is get as much sunshine as possible. The sun activates hundreds of genes – vitamin D is only one benefit but it's a big one. Forget about sunscreen – sunscreen itself seems to be causing melanomas after the skin soaks up the strong chemicals and the immune system has yet another battle on its hands. Just use your own sense of when enough is enough – and maybe wear a hat!

10. Coconut oil butter – A great find is using coconut oil butter instead of margarine. One teaspoon of

margarine has enough useless, suffocating saturated fat molecules to provide 50,000 of them to every cell in your body. On the other hand, the coconut (cold pressed, organic only) product has medium chain fatty acids which neurons can also use as a source of energy. It survives heating, so can be used for cooking.

11. Visualisation – has been strongly linked to extended survival in cancer patients, and this ties in with the work of Bruce Lipton (also referred to in Marilyn Bennett's story). Lipton was a genetic scientist. He theorised that it was the environment created by the individual which was damaging the cell, as there was nothing wrong with the cell itself. Consequently, why the emotional environment is so critical to recovery, something my father, a haematologist, noticed from his work more than two decades ago. Dr Joanna Budwig herself noticed her therapies didn't work on women who remained in abusive marriages. This alarming idea tells you something important about the roots of disorder in our bodies, and something useful about the immune system – do what makes you happy!

12. Go Natural – Rather than getting a kick from coffee which ruins your pH and produces a lethargic and addictive coming down period, go natural.

13. Exercise – Another thing you can do is get to the gym: after you start imbibing vegetables and dumping processed foods you find yourself with more energy. After exercise, the additional resources the muscles consume mean less to feed the tumour.

14. Sleep – Following the natural hours of sleep allows the body to heal faster.

15. Yoga – And only last week I started some yoga lessons – this is great for expanding and stretching the limbs to help the lymphatic system. The teacher is talented and very patient, the class very accepting of one who has the flexibility of a brick, and the room is calm and quiet. The world stands still for an hour while, amidst like minds, you get to grips with your own self. Now that's what I call a prescription!

Leaving the cause in place

Yesterday I went for a check-up at Bedford Hospital's ENT department. I met with the two surgeons most familiar with my case, who always gently recommend chemotherapy and radiation, which I, equally gently, always refuse. This time they both observed that the outstanding tumour on my neck was definitely smaller. I have to be honest: it doesn't matter how rebellious you might be or how into natural therapies and alternative medicine, the authority of experienced, serious doctors is deeply ingrained. Despite myself, their words filled me with renewed confidence. Before every appointment I consider cancelling, partly out of fear, but I go anyway because I enjoy their company. Like me, they are looking for answers, and I just happen to be caught in the middle as both experimenter and experiment. I feel that, if I can convince them, I must have nothing to worry about. Being open minded, one took notes about my vegetable juice regimen, including watercress – which prevents tumours co-opting new blood supplies – and lemons, which raise the pH. After hearing how I abandoned my extreme coffee habit he seemed concerned about his own habit of ten cups a day, perhaps more so after seeing me bound into the surgery, down to the same weight as when I was eighteen, without a sniff of caffeine in a year.

Half-jokingly, I asked if they thought any surgeon anywhere would – for a modest fee – just excise the lump and send me on my way. I was told in no uncertain terms this would contravene every medical principle in the book: treating one tumour in isolation from the original, giving the patient a false sense of security while leaving their fate unchanged. I was assured they would personally report such a doctor if they ever found out his name, and get him debarred. No doubt they were right, and deep down I agreed, though I still think it's worth asking. But only when driving home I realised that the position should actually be broader still. Currently medicine treats tumours (even as a networked group) in *isolation* from the *true cause,* that is, the tissue milieu from which they grew – and will grow again in the future – from a predictable need to survive adverse conditions. This milieu provides their opportunity once the immune system, closely woven with the mind, becomes overburdened or distracted. Without question, in fifty years cancer will not be treated in this way – assaulting the tumour with chemicals and radiation while leaving *the person* unchanged; giving them hope of a cure while leaving the cause in place.

There's no such thing as bad publicity

Last week I put the finishing touches on my house fresco. As I'd suspected, those who had commented loudly on the scaffolding's extended presence could hardly remember it being there only two days later. I was invited to talk on the radio. A charming reporter from

ITV turned up and in no time flat absorbed the technicalities and recorded enough film to put together a concise piece which appeared on TV only three hours later, hitting the coveted 10:00 pm national news slot: http://www.itv.com/news/anglia/update/2014-06-11/meet-the-man-from-bedford-whos-paintedafresco-on-the-side-of-his-house/

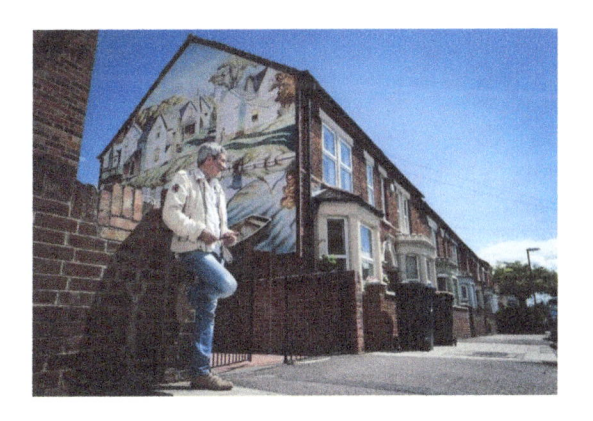

A little advice

So keep positive, think of the best, believe in yourself, and stay well!

'Finally, brethren, whatsoever things are true, whatsoever things are honest, whatsoever things are just, whatsoever things are pure, whatsoever things are lovely, whatsoever things are of good report; if there be any virtue, and if there be any praise, think on these things'.

Philippians 4:8

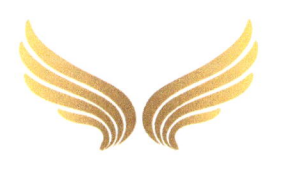

"I am now flying and free of the chains that had been holding me down. Life is exciting".

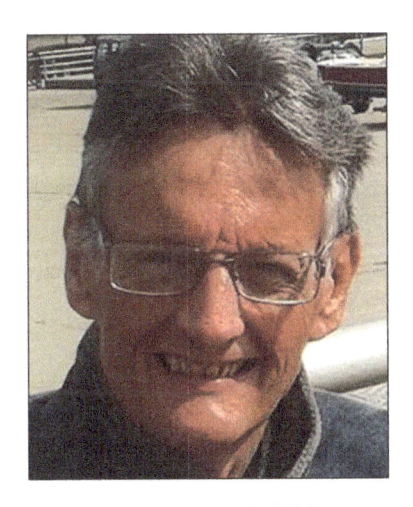

GORDON ROSS

Gordon 'touched' me through my good friend Robin Daly of Yes to Life Charity in London. I telephoned Gordon and listened humbly to his challenging, transforming story of healing on all levels. Gordon's strong faith throughout his cancer, led him on an amazing journey of discovery and healing. It's almost like his faith propels him out of himself, empowering him to see things in a new light – a new light that is to lead him down a very different path!

Here Gordon shares his healing with you:

It was to be a moment that shook me to the core. I was driving between jobs from Melton Mowbray to Leicester some time in 1998. The road was dry and the visibility good. Suddenly I had a flat tyre: you know that monotonous bumping sound on one side of the car? Yes, definitely a flat tyre...no question. I pulled over and looked at the wheel in question... no flat tyre, no soft tyre...in fact a perfect tyre; indeed all the tyres were perfect. Very strange! I looked back up the road for some bumps, a poor road surface....nothing ...I was really bemused. I got back in the car after a minute had passed and started up again ...the car was running perfectly. A few hundred yards along, I glanced at a group of 6 or so young children cycling along the road going the other way. A few hundred yards later the road took a sharp left bend and that's when the voice went off inside my head. It was loud and clear: "This is where you would have hit the children....!" I pulled over in a sweat. I had to think this through....I started to think how long I had been delayed by stopping and how far I would have travelled in that time. Wow! It was starting to sink in. I was just comprehending that the time and distance fitted pretty well. Somehow, either the children or I, or both, had been supernaturally saved from a collision. I also knew instinctively that God had arranged the delay, in order to protect me and others around me.

Now let me say right away that I am a logical sort of guy. I'm a structural engineer. I deal with numbers, science, rules and facts. I have enjoyed most of my working life, the maths of design and construction of large public structures. Having said that, for as long as I can remember, I have been fascinated by people, their mannerisms, and their body language. Understanding what they really mean when they say something and display their body habits, and all that sort of stuff. I am conscious that a specific solution or advice matches the individual client. I am far from the art side of life. It's more or less been 'Facts and Science' for me.

I was hit to my knees with an electricity- like force so powerful

When our only son was born in 1995, I, or rather we, thought it was the decent thing to have him baptized, to which our vicar surprised us by agreeing to do the deed without reservation. So he had said "Yes, no catches" but he asked my wife and I to think of joining an Alpha Course, which is a non-believers' starter course to Christianity. I thought: the vicar's been good to us; he has agreed to the baptism, so we will agree to go to a couple of evenings of this course and we pack it in and the deal is done. I have always liked a deal: something for something, a trade. Everybody is then happy. Well, to cut a long story short, I became really intrigued by the course but was especially interested in the testimony of one man who seemed to be able to not offend the very simplistic thought processes of an engineer such as myself. I carried on, I went to the weekend away on the course and I found myself challenging God to prove Himself. I wasn't going to accept a theoretical presence. I needed to know if God was real, and to do this, I had to be sure He knows me in person. I needed proof and I wanted it now, or I was walking away from this whole business. On reflection now an outrageous request, but there you have it. I caught up with the vicar and told him what I was thinking. He asked if there was any sin in my life that needed discussing. No, I just need to know God. He put his hand on my head, said a prayer. Nothing happened for about a minute. I was just beginning to feel a little foolish with this fellow's palm on my head, when I was hit to my knees with an electricity like force so powerful, I was in tears but realised this was God showing me what He means to me, an Amazing Power. I found myself acknowledging Jesus Christ as my Saviour and begging His forgiveness for doubting His reality. A few words later and I was born again, that is to say, I had welcomed Jesus Christ and the Holy Spirit into my life. Very dramatic it was too. I had dared to challenge God and He had given me what I had wanted, the proof. Tracking forward, I had an amazing time for about 18 months. I ran Alpha Courses for people enquiring about Jesus Christ. I also managed the project of building a 2 story extension to my church. I designed a new mezzanine floor for another church. God was right in there, helping me with the funding, dealing with contractors and I was really enjoying myself. It was Holy Spirit fun. There were a number of experiences of the Holy Spirit that either helped me get out of tricky corners or encouraged me in some way. However, in hindsight, I had no-one to help me keep the fire burning inside me. I would eventually succumb to all the classic worldly trappings.

Within 2 years of living with God's Spirit, all the fun had died and the buzz had gone. My spiritual experiences were firmly pushed into the past. I had become very judgemental of folk at church, and especially the leaders who I viewed as definitely not holy and some of them quite manipulative. It was as if the closer I got to people, the less I liked what I saw. Not what I had expected at all and it beat me up terribly. I left the church and soon after, my wife and I moved to Torquay in Devon in order to enjoy a less pacey lifestyle. Indeed, we have enjoyed a number of years living in a beautiful coastal bay. What could be more restful, a place by the sea and a job without too much stress...I had suffered from minor bouts of depression on and off for years. All this would hopefully be behind me for good.

The warning signs had started as early as 2002. I had been diagnosed with Type 2 diabetes, which I initially tried to deal with through what I perceived as an improved diet. Despite my half-hearted attempts, I couldn't stick to a serious routine so I eventually ended on medication for, not just the diabetes, but also high blood pressure and also the dreaded statins for the alleged control of cholesterol, which was never a problem for me anyway. We moved to Torquay in 2005 in order to improve our lifestyle and reduce the work stress levels. It was certainly a good move with great potential, but my old ways were to creep slowly back into my life. I decided that I wouldn't find a church yet. I would get settled in to our new home and job at the Local Authority offices. I would, in time go back to church, or so I thought, without doing much about it. Anyway, despite the varied and enjoyable work, the bouts of workplace stress and depression came back. After 7 or so years in Torquay, I was also drinking very heavily to wipe out the stress at work. Working relationships were poor within the workplace with a lot of personal issues between individuals and poor management of the situations. Many of my colleagues had little or no experience of working outside of a Local Authority environment and did not adapt well to a culture of change. Like most men in my situation, I still didn't hear or see the alarm bells, I just pushed them to one side.

The roof finally fell in on me

The roof finally fell in on me on October 17th 2012. My life stopped when, after choking on some food, my good wife suggested I see the doctor who sent me for an endoscopy down my eating tube, "Just to be safe", she said. There on the hospital bed, it all came crashing in on me. The tumour was so invasive; the technician could not push the endoscope past the tumour just above the stomach. It was so big. "I am so sorry to tell you, Mr Ross, it would seem you have an advanced tumour in your oesophagus….".Yes, your life flies in front of you. I can't have a tumour, I'm a fit guy……oh no you aren't, Gordon, I start to think. The warning signs, the diabetes, the stress, the alcohol….and now it's too late… isn't it. I am going to die.

Two weeks of mayhem followed. I was sent for scans, investigations down my breathing tube and around the stomach with the result that I was told the tumour was 50mm long and also extended into the stomach. It was between stage 3 and 4, stage 4 being the highest level. Surgery was ruled out of the question as there were too many enlarged lymph nodes all over my body. The general stomach appearance didn't look good either, despite the tumour being limited to the upper part of the stomach wall. I remember having a strange sense of relief. I didn't want to lose my stomach anyway; I wanted to keep my body. Well, I got my wish: no surgery, but

I was eventually offered palliative chemo that would keep me "as comfortable as possible" for up to 2 years. At the end of this period, I was told I would die.

Around this time, the first of my "Angels" appeared on the scene. Tony turned up at the golf course bar one evening after I had finished playing a round and after a brief introduction, he suggested I go to see Dr Stephen Hopwood at the Arcturus Cancer Care Clinic in Totnes. Stephen had been a great help to him with a cancer in his pituitary gland. I thought, what is there to lose? So off I went and this is where I really started my journey. I would meet with Stephen weekly for about a year, during which times I would learn about the drivers of cancer, what may have caused my cancer, what I can do about the illness and the options available to me, both clinical and natural. He assured me I had time to consider my options. He would give me acupuncture, and also recommended a whole range of supplements and an alkalised diet guide. I recall thinking at this point: Stephen Hopwood is making sense to me. I have been responsible for allowing my body to become cancerous, so I need to take responsibility for my healing. I need help to do this; I need to build a team around me that is up for the challenge. I started to change my lifestyle completely. I gave up alcohol, wheat, dairy products, red meats and started to work out what I could actually eat, which was not easy! This change was very difficult as it had a huge impact on not just me but also on my family. I was, however, surprised at how easily I gave up alcohol, which had been such a prop. I was to grow in due course not only to avoid alcohol but actually to dislike its taste. For a Scot brought up on whisky and heavy (beer), this was a revelation for me as I had a secret thought I may at one point have been an alcoholic. Deciding to remove all diabetic related medication from my body, I was in battle mode to find out if a radical regime could change my health.

I was making an improvement in my life in a brand new way

I attended an alternative cancer conference in November 2012, and two things gripped me. One, I could not understand the language of the alternative therapists. They spoke of cancer in a way I just could not comprehend, especially the holistic stuff. Secondly, there were people there who spoke in very simple language. I remember a retired GP speaking about diabetes as a forerunner to cancer... gulp! He also spoke about diabetics needing to research the particular carbohydrate that is abnormally raising their sugar levels as a norm, thus making them susceptible to the effects of sugar spikes in their blood. This fascinated me as it was something I could potentially do to make a difference. I went home, determined to find out if what he said was true. I tested my blood sugar readings immediately after a number of foods (meals were slow to complete at that time). It didn't take me long to find out what was raising my sugar level abnormally. It was potato, boiled, roasted fried, it mattered not. I had been eating potato all my life in many forms and it was the culprit all along. I tested other carbohydrates but they weren't having a similar adverse impact on me. I was so happy; I was making an improvement in my life in a brand new way. I cut out potato from my diet. Just like that! It was easy.

I had lots of questions about the cancer inside me. How big was it? What is its form? How far did it extend into my body? What were its cells made of....? All sorts of questions. Whenever I met oncologists, not only would I not get good answers, I was being dissuaded from asking the questions in the first place. I was, in effect, being told to trust them as my best option, just because they were doctors! My brain was telling me I was being fobbed off. My brain has always had a distrustful eye for the 'trust me, I know what I'm doing' routine. I have always pushed the specialist in any walk of life to explain their actions to me in words I can understand. Indeed, just as I have sought to do for others. The 'trust me' routine was coming at me time after time and it was getting smelly. I was actually told that I shouldn't be asking such questions; that I should leave it to the experts. This only served to make me even more suspicious and wondering where the truth lies. I went to London for a second opinion and was told the same stuff: accept my fate that I would eventually die and, in the meantime, accept palliative chemo. Something that the London doctor told me that really antagonised me was him telling me, in desperation to get me out of his office, that it was probably too late for me anyway. I told him he was a disgrace; he threw me out. I will never forget those words. They didn't depress me, they only served to light a spark in me to find the truth of my cancer and to beat this enemy.

Served to light a spark in me
At the time I was so angry. On the train journey home, I encountered a young couple just starting off in married life. They opened up, asking me all sorts of stuff about

what to do about financial stuff and how to deal with other people including family. I found myself helping them with my experience of life. I would continue in my search for the truth about cancer as I had much to offer and I really enjoyed the banter of meeting others. I also knew I wanted to be part of my son's life as he was soon to embark on university life.

Back home again, I knew that what I was doing was making a difference and I achieved a success only a couple of months after starting my new eating and drinking regime (minus potato). I had my six monthly diabetic check and my HP1AC levels had dramatically dropped from 65 to 28. Wow! I was making a difference to my health in a way I could never have imagined. Success! I was no longer diabetic. I also knew this would help me in my cancer battle. There was another strong pull on me at that time and it was getting stronger by the day. I made the decision that I needed to go back and unashamedly seek God in this mess. I remember all those years earlier, describing myself to my vicar in Loughborough as a Prodigal Son that needed to be let go. I soon left the Church. Despite all my failings, I was being reminded that if God is as good as his word, he would welcome me back. The amazing thing about the choice of church to go to wasn't really a choice. It had already been determined for me many years earlier.

"Go to that church!"
Sixteen years earlier I had been on holiday with my wife in Torquay, soon after I had been met by God's Holy Spirit. I recall driving down a road in Torquay and God's

voice in my head saying: "*Go to that Church*" ...I just continued on the road, ignoring the voice. The same thing happened the following day. As I drove past the church, God's voice again said "Go to That Church". This time I decided to accede and I duly attended the following Sunday. I had a reassuring experience during the proceedings where at one point I was pinned to the pew, lying full length, unable to move with God telling me: "I knew you in Loughborough, I know you in Torquay, I know you wherever you are". Not unpleasant, I thought, reassuring, but otherwise the event had no other meaning for me at the time.

"It's who you are NOW that matters."

Little did I know that I was to walk into the same church all those years later. I was pretty distraught by now. I was improving my diet but what if wasn't enough? I was being told by the experts that there was nothing I could do to avoid dying of cancer. What could God do about this? I was made very welcome at Riviera Life Church. It was very different to the proceedings 16 years earlier: certainly, much busier. After about 3 weeks of meeting new friends and telling them of my predicament, I was taken aback to hear God's voice again after all those years in the wilderness. I was in the bath at home one evening, and I was praying: "God, I don't want to die. I want to live because I want to serve you." A response came back at me immediately: "Don't you realise that you already serve me!" It was amazing to hear his voice again. The words were just as Jesus would admonish his disciples, "Don't you realise, Gordon...? Haven't you worked it out yet...? It's not what you are aspiring to be that matters; it's who you are NOW that matters." This was a revelation for me. It was the first confirmation that I wasn't finished, that I was serving my God right now, in the midst of all this confusion and condemnation. What an encouragement for me! It was also a warning not to feel sorry for myself nor to blame others for my predicament but to be patient (not my natural way) and look to help others now, not at some point in the future.

After discussing with my family and Stephen, I decided to go for the palliative chemotherapy. What I appreciated particularly was him directly challenging my motives thoroughly until he was satisfied. I had thought it through properly. This is the first time I started to understand the importance of fully articulating your motives and wishes in your speech as you confirm the thoughts in your head. This was to prove a revelation time and time again on my journey. I saw the palliative chemotherapy as a means to eventually be healed, once I discovered my next steps after this therapy. At the time, it was so reassuring to have someone without an agenda to bounce my thoughts, fears and intentions. Once we were clear on the reasons for chemotherapy, he recommended a number of supplements and Chinese chemo support herbal teas that he believed would help protect my vital organs from the ravages of chemotherapy.

It was somewhere around this time, I began to receive phone calls and visits from folk offering support, many of whom I had never previously been close to. The other more disquieting experience that was happening was that some of the folk I had been close to were awfully quiet when they learned of my situation. Some of these folk would actually soon avoid me in the street, when I was able to get out between chemo poundings. This upset me for some time. Eventually, I came to realise that it wasn't me they were avoiding but the cancer. In prayer time, I was realising that God was starting me off on a journey of forgiving an awful lot of folk who would not support me for whatever reason. When they heard the word 'terminal', they really believed it! Not for me!

I was there to be shot at

This business I spoke about earlier about getting to know the experts close up and not liking what I saw, was beginning to pay off to my advantage. I didn't accept the expert view of terminal cancer because they were not explaining their thoughts in a clear rational manner, nor were they taking the time to understand me or the cancer inside me. As I stepped out from the crowd, I was there to be shot at for having an enquiring mind and determination to get to the truth of cancer. I had to forgive certain friends and family for their attitude towards me but at the same time move them to one side for the foreseeable future. I needed positivity around me and I was determined to understand fully ALL the reasons for the cancer and eliminate the source. I was certain that harbouring grudges with others was not going to help me one bit.

No-one who has gone through the standard four cycles, let alone eight cycles of EOX chemotherapy I went through, needs me to tell them the devastating impact of this treatment on the body. I won't go into detail but it's not pleasant and nothing can prepare you for what you feel like and become at its most severe. After six cycles, I actually felt a bit better. I recall asking questions regarding the chemotherapy success and once again all I received was vague references to some improvement in the tumour size. No definitive success statements, but there again if I knew then how it had benefited me I would only have been encouraged to press on challenging the NHS to complete the cure. I remember thinking; all this effort to get through this devastating therapy and all I am getting is vague comments. As I was feeling better, I was becoming more determined to find answers to push on with more solutions. I was beginning to pick up my energy and also my brain was not so fuzzy. I would also go to church once every three weeks, whenever I was recovering between each cycle.

"I lifted you up today!"

On one of those occasions at church, another amazing thing happened to me. I was praising God (as normal) and I suddenly had a sense of being lifted up into the air. Physically, I was still on the ground but spiritually and with my eyes wide open I was able to look down on the congregation with my head at about 12 foot or so in the air. It was a thrilling experience and I was certainly enjoying myself as I looked down watching others praising God with their hands raised. After about 30 seconds or so, I dropped back down. Now this was new to me. I had heard of people with 'out of body' experiences, but this was difficult for me to understand. Soon after I had 'landed' and was wondering what had just happened, the lady next to me asked" What happened to you?" I said I didn't know and I asked her what she saw. She said that I had a look of wonder on my face for the time I had experienced being lifted up. I was intrigued by it

all but had no real answers. By that evening I had forgotten all about what happened, and I was again enjoying my regular Epsom salts bath. As I relaxed, I heard God's voice again: "I lifted you up today!" I responded "You've got my attention all right". Again, the voice came back at me: "I want you to sit on my shoulders so that you can see things you have never been able to see before" .....
Well, this really rocked my boat. Tears pouring down my face, I was remembering how, at five years old, my natural father would lift me on his shoulders every night when he came home from work and paraded me down the street outside. I was amazed at what I could see from that height and I loved it. My spiritual Father was now demonstrating to me some amazing truths. For one, He knows me so well and knows what I like. Secondly, He has so much wisdom to share with me. Thirdly, there is no way all this spiritual experience was going to be wasted on me. I was certain at that point I was going to live. I was buzzing with confidence. I also sensed all I had to do now was to work out how to make it happen.

My oncologist tried to persuade me to end the systemic chemotherapy after four cycles then, after the maximum of six cycles. Me, being the determined type, and as I had committed to this therapy, I was determined to see it through until my body wanted to end the treatment. I held out for eight cycles and got them. By the end of seven cycles my body was telling me: "One more and that's it". I was beginning to tire of the treatment.

I received £15,002 in just 6 weeks.
As I have previously explained, despite my oncologist thinking I would decline, like many others from here on

on, I saw the systemic chemotherapy as a step in the road to recovery. I started researching outside of the NHS with the help of Dr Hopwood. I spoke with Patricia Peat at Cancer Options in Mansfield after going via a cancer charity called YES TO LIFE, based in London. One of the options she spoke of was a Doctor in Germany called Professor Thomas Vogl based at the University Hospital in Frankfurt. He had an embolised chemotherapy that could possibly be an option for me. I researched him on the internet and really became interested in his techniques. Alas, the money needed was out of my reach. At about £4500 for each visit including hotels and flights, I could not afford such sums. In stepped my next Angel. I had met Andrew, who had liver cancer, earlier on my journey in a hyperbaric chamber in Exeter and we became instant friends. We had since gone off on our own treatment journeys. Here he was now sitting next to me in my local hospital as I was receiving my seventh cycle of chemotherapy. He was having a blood transfusion after his first trip to Frankfurt to see Professor Vogl. It was a conversation that was Spirit-led. It was amazing. Andrew was full of praise for the treatment and he also told me how to raise the money needed for my treatment. Ask friends and colleagues via the 'Just Giving' website and 'YES TO LIFE', who receive the money on your behalf give you the money back on receipt of proof of spending. Simple! ..... Ah, not quite....asking people for money, not for me, never done that, far too proud for that..... It took me a week of soul searching and eventually I changed my mind. I wrote out my story so far, set up the web page and went live, sending the link to about seventy people that I knew well enough to ask them to help me. I thought, if I get enough for one treatment, I could borrow the rest and maybe we could manage. I targeted £15,000 for the 3 treatments that Professor Vogl told me I would need and waited. It didn't take long. I was stunned by the response from people I knew and others who had my story forwarded to them. I received £15,002 in just 6 weeks. My former church in Loughborough had even found out about my plight and gave a sizeable sum to close the total target. I was being blessed again by God. I was amazed at how generous people could be.

My wife and I went off to Frankfurt and the first good news we received was that, after his first MRI scan, the Professor told me that he would treat me, that his target was my healing and he even showed me the size of the tumour on his MRI scan. He was answering clinical questions to which I was never previously receiving satisfactory answers. I was very happy and my spirit was soaring. He told me that my tumour had been reduced to about 10mm in size by the 8 cycles of chemotherapy. The UK chemotherapy had helped me feel better but it could not finish the job off. Hence, this may well be why you don't get to know too much of the detail of partial healing. After three treatments on my tumour and two key lymph nodes, he wanted to give me more treatments to turn a large area of pre- cancer cells, the size of two tennis balls around the tumour back into to healthy cells again. I could see this was going to take many more than three trips to get the all clear.

What I wish for, I will receive!
It was to be the best decision on my part that I have ever made on this journey. It was done with the help of

another Angel. It concerned the necessary finance to complete the treatment. I sat down and discussed a lot of 'what ifs' with a friend who was really into financial options and out popped the answer. It was brilliant. The system had me as terminal, so I would use this status to my advantage. I decided to retire from my employment, with my pension fund increasing my retirement pot to the level it would be if I were 65 years old. I would use the pension lump sum to pay off both the mortgage on our house but, more importantly, finance the remaining treatments. Brilliant! What a great move! In one fell swoop I would eliminate the source of my workplace stress and deal with my immediate financial needs at the same time. This allowed me to complete five further embolised chemotherapy treatments and also a laser treatment to burn the remains of the tumour. The laser treatment was astounding as to its audacity. Way ahead of anything in the UK. I won't go into detail as it could frighten some folk. Safe to say, it's a procedure that Professor Vogl does not get to use on all patients as it's a final "wipe out" of the remains once the tumour has been shrunk to a very small size indeed. I was sitting in his Frankfurt Hospital reception when the Professor came up to me and sat by me to have my signature on the procedure forms before the laser treatment. I continue to be amazed by this man: what doctor in the UK would sit by your side in a waiting room? Not many, I suspect. Anyway, I signed the form and he said to me casually: "Fingers Crossed, Mr Ross!" After asking him to repeat that statement, I said: "I'm not crossing any fingers, because that means I have no confidence in the man sitting next to me, for you are the best man I could be sitting next to right now." He smiled, nodded and went off to prepare for the procedure. German humour or testing me? I was now completely in the zone of understanding the importance of the words I speak in relation to what my mind is thinking. It's also about integrity in the moment. I was now convinced that what I wish for, I will receive. This has been an important lesson. I am not capable of thinking one thing and saying another at the same time. So I understood, right there and then, that my immediate positive response to the professor was also deep within my spirit. I was confident of my healing, simply because of my immediate response to him. This has proved to be a huge lesson for me as I move out of this illness. Be careful of what you say because it reflects your innermost belief. What a revelation!

During the summer of 2014, I was invited to attend a Christian conference on the Isle of Wight. The way I was invited also made me suspect that God had something special to say to me. Anyway, I really appreciated the pastor who was running the event, rather than the invited speaker. On the final afternoon, I insisted on saying goodbye to him. I had never previously met this chap and we only spoke briefly during the event, but he proceeded to tell me some very personal things about my character. Specifically, he told me that I was a square peg in a round hole and that I would never be completely comfortable in the company of any one group; that I constantly needed to meet new people and this is not a matter by which I should consider myself inadequate or limited in any way. It's just the way it has to be with me. Now this assessment has my character spot on. My history with church hierarchy and my fascination with the characteristics of people make this journey all the more surprising. More work in progress in this area I suspect.

The Holy Spirit inside me roared like a lion

Two things started to happen involving others: firstly, people started to hear that I was making good progress with my own health and were hearing of someone with the determination not to accept the condemnation of a terminal illness. I did a video testimony at the 'YES TO LIFE' offices in March 2014 in which my story was encouraging others to press on with their journey of healing, despite the negativity of clinicians in the UK. I was getting calls from people from different parts of the UK, from people who were being referred to me, requesting me to tell them my story. When I finished talking to them, I would also pray for their healing in the name of Jesus.

Now while all this is going on, I found myself becoming very interested in the work of a pastor from the USA called Curry Blake. Curry leads the John G Lake Ministries in Texas. His teachings have been making the New Testament Bible ever more clear for me whilst slaying the rules and ceremonies that man has put into the Christian faith over the centuries. Curry argues that all Christian believers who have the Holy Spirit inside of them can, and should, be healing others with illnesses with the authority of Jesus. I was watching his 17 videos on YouTube over a two week period and becoming really captivated as to how simple the Christian faith should be. Near the end of the last video, the Holy Spirit inside me roared like a lion for about a minute or so. Was this God's approval of Curry Blake, a sign for me, or indeed my healing taking place? I know not yet, but what it did do is give me the encouragement to command that all sickness be removed from the bodies of people I encounter. Now, this is clearly not possible in my own strength, but with God's guidance I started to be confident to simply touch people lightly and command their illness to leave in the name of Jesus. I have started getting results, and I am determined to press on in this work. There is a lot more to experience and to learn here.

I did have had one set back on my journey which did knock me at the time. In April 2014, I travelled back to Loughborough to meet lots of folk who had supported me financially. I was feeling good and had energy but I realise now that my body's adrenalin was compensating for a limited amount of energy. Within 4 days of bounding around meeting folk and doing testimonies at 2 churches in the town, I was hit with Bell's palsy. This is an infection of a facial gland in front of the ear. My speech, balance, hearing, sight, taste and smell were all battered and I could not use any of my senses. I found the next 6 weeks very frustrating as there was nothing I could do at all. This frightened me, but there is one thing I did learn and that is to respect my body, to appreciate rest times, and to say "YES" when help is offered. Six months later and there are still some small feelings of the Palsy but most of the visual impact on my face has gone. Respect for my body from now on!

I have recently been celebrating the anniversary of my cancer diagnosis on 17th October 2012, when I was given up to two years to live. I am alive and very much kicking those who haven't got the point that healing of the mind, body and spirit are all connected and need attention. I know that full and permanent healing is not possible for one without the other two. I was asked by a friend when we were enjoying the anniversary, what 3 things would I recommend to him in order to avoid contracting cancer. My immediate response was:

1. Avoid long term stress in your life i.e. in the region of two years or so. I believe short term stress has positive benefits but not stress that you cannot overcome. My wholehearted recommendation to beat debilitating stress is by committing to a life-long faith in Christ, and a daily relationship with The Holy Spirit.
2. Avoid dietary excesses, in particular processed food, alcohol and the big S ... Sugar. These are huge drivers for cancers. A healthy balanced diet of low level meats and plenty of vegetables with plenty of regular exercise will keep most cancers at bay.
3. Always look to do something out of the box. An exciting activity, meeting up with people, helping others, making an effort to go into an area that is against your natural thinking process. The results are amazing!

I am in remission from the cancer. Professor Vogl tells me *there is no cancer activity in my body* and my first MRI screening in Frankfurt is due next month, in November 2014. My local NHS will not scan me any more as I am not in agreement to any more systemic chemotherapy. I have been back in part time employment for the last six months, working part time on a zero hours' contract for a friend. I am enjoying my work in providing structural advice and solutions for people for whom I enjoy working. They are generally thankful for my efforts. What could be simpler?

I am now flying

What I say and what I believe is so interconnected and has been a strong driver in my healing. Being careful (and with integrity) in what I say, impacts very strongly on my beliefs and consequently on how I am feeling in terms of my health. This is another area for me to understand more deeply. My journey has, and continues, to amaze me. Through this illness and my experiences of his protective and caring ways, I know that God is willing to give me what I want, not just what I need. These are two very different things. What I needed was full healing. What I wanted was to take responsibility for dealing with the illness. I had allowed all these horrible things to get into my life and I desired ownership of the healing process. I believe I have rejected the evil drivers of the cancer forever. Like the good Father He is, God has let me take charge, as far I could understand the responsibility for my healing. He put Angels and the Holy Spirit in place to keep me on the healing path. Amazing! I just want to keep close to Him to know more of His goodness.

I am now flying and free of the chains that had been holding me down. Life is exciting. My sincere apologies to all the angels I have not mentioned. I had to stop at some point.

A little advice

1. *When diagnosed, don't panic. Most people have time to put a plan together. You are now number one on your priority list: it's all about what <u>you</u> want from now on in.*

2. *Get hold of at least one person who is knowledgeable and trustworthy who can act as a cancer life coach with whom you can to talk through everything and anything. Most importantly, try to work out why you have cancer. This will help you immensely on your journey.*

3. *Don't commit to any treatment just because someone said you should do it. Do it because it either makes sense to you or it actually makes you feel better emotionally or physically (or both).*

4. *Don't submit to any person. I recommend you have your faith only in Jesus Christ. Find a Christian Church that relates to you and declares that it's God's will to heal you.*

5. *Don't stress about getting everything right at the beginning. It's a journey where you come across people and treatments along the road. Some you take on board, others you have to discard for the journey. Value those people who come to you and stay with you for the duration of your journey.*

6. *Celebrate every little success. Discard any news or person who says you can't do anything about the cancer. It's a massive lie. Seek to live only in truth.*

My Prayer for Your Healing

Finally, I am sending a prayer to anyone reading this chapter who has cancer: "I declare you to have life, full health and be free of all sickness and spirits of sickness, in the name of Jesus Christ. Amen".

'I had to go forward from here'

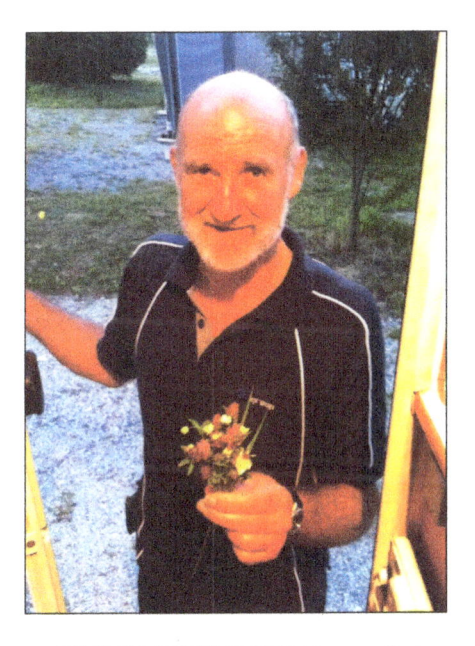

GLENN JOHNSON (Australia)

Glenn and I connected indirectly as it were. My friend Pauline whose chapter appears later, upon hearing that I was amazed by Marilyn's story, suggested that I should definitely hear her partner Glenn's remarkable journey. I emailed Marilyn's son Steven in Australia, and he willingly agreed that Glenn his dad, would be more than happy for me to include his story, which I have encapsulated here with input from Marilyn throughout. All the way through Glenn's story I could see how important it was to him that Marilyn was by his side and often at the forefront of his treatment choices and decisions.

Here Glenn shares his courageous story:

Why me?
This is the first big question a person generally asks when confronted with a medical diagnosis that we have the big C. What did I do to deserve this? What did I do wrong? And the myriad of other questions that follow. Stress, excess alcohol consumption and smoking have been highlighted as possible causes of oesophageal carcinoma. In my case, the above could be construed as being the underlying factors that may have had some sort of influence in my being diagnosed with cancer. No mention that nutrition (or lack of correct nutrition) could have contributed to this. What about the amount of water a person consumes over the years?

I would have sworn otherwise
Previous to this incident, my health had been excellent with only an odd cold or flu to bother me or a broken bone or two, which, to me, is part of life and entirely acceptable. I thought that I was relatively indestructible and did not have any thought of succumbing to a serious health problem when I was first diagnosed. There was no history of cancer in the family. I did take up the habits of smoking and drinking alcohol at an early age like my father. I didn't last too long at smoking as I watched my father surrender to emphysema over a long period and I was somehow wise enough to realize the adverse effects of smoking. At that stage, I was in my early twenties (thirty odd years ago). As drinking was/is a social interaction and was widely accepted as some macho thing, I was not going to be left out of the crowd. Beer was the main form of alcohol I consumed. I did cut back on my drinking habits as I got older and wiser (and the effects of too much alcohol took longer to get over).

I did not consider, rightly or wrongly, that I was an alcoholic. I married and divorced during this period. I still enjoy a wine or two daily. About ten years ago, I did add spirits to my fairly average beer consumption (three to four standard drinks) as a before bed toddy. A good shot or two of whisky make you sleep better, so they say. Had my brief stint at smoking or my rather full-on alcohol intake have any direct effect on my getting cancer? I don't really know.

As most of us are aware, stress affects different people in different ways. Recently, I have come to realize that I have been somewhat susceptible to stress during my life though I would have sworn otherwise. Mood swings, rather quick to anger, (though it did not last long) some sleepless nights, and several other indicators which I can now relate to stress level increases. Maybe this susceptibility was inherent or through work influences or by other means. I did run my own labour hire business for about four years some fifteen years ago but, more recently through choice, have been working as a health and safety professional for major construction contractors. This position certainly has its ups and downs. My work has been generally deskbound so, to maintain my fitness levels, I exercised fairly regularly by indulging in rowing, swimming, cycling and walking. Stress, was it a factor in my situation? Again I (and they) don't really know. I have always had an excellent relationship with my partner Marilyn, so relationship-stress was not a contributing factor, as far as I was concerned.

"I beg your pardon, what did you say?"
There we were, a few weeks out from going on an island holiday, when I believe I first experienced the symptoms

that would take us on this epic journey. I had an acute indigestion attack that lasted several hours. I put that down to something I ate or drank, as one would with little knowledge of the internal workings of the body. Over the next week or two, I experienced at least one similar condition with intermittent reflux (burping and heartburn). Again I thought this was a simple indigestive thing. Not an unusual occurrence for someone my age. At last, off we went on our holiday. Nothing was going to spoil this break and at that stage I certainly was not really concerned with or had any inkling as to the implications of these minor bouts of annoyance.

During the holiday, I started suffering an increase in indigestion, reflux and lower chest pain. I did not seem to have any difficulties swallowing then. I kept these symptoms to myself so as not to take the enjoyment out of our holiday. I did resolve to see my local doctor when we arrived back home. Not long after our return, I made an appointment with my local doctor. I had been going to him for several years and respected his skills and knowledge. I explained my symptoms. He recommended I attend a hospital for an endoscopy. I made the appointment within two weeks.

On my way home from work two days later, I had a phone call from my doctor requesting I visit his surgery and obtain the results of the procedure. My doctor explained in a professional manner that I had a carcinoma in the oesophagus. "I beg your pardon, what did you say?" The doctor repeated the statement and I blurted out: 'You mean to say I have the Big C!' I was shown the report. Just the sight of the photo sent shivers down my spine. I didn't expect this result. The information did not compute for a moment or two. This could not relate to me. I felt a sinking feeling in the pit of my stomach. Being naïve as I was on the outcomes of anyone who is diagnosed with any form of cancer, my first thought was that this was the end of the road. Was this a dream? No, this was 5.00pm on a Friday afternoon. My scattered mind was trying to focus. Where do I go from here? My doctor knew a good surgeon in this field. Within minutes, my doctor had contacted the surgeon and arranged for me to visit him the following week. My feet had not touched the ground and I was already caught up in the system. I did not know any better and thought this was my only option. I left with my head in a haze and agonizing where my life was heading from that day. Yes, I did ask myself all the questions on why, how, what and so on. The diagnosis came as a shock, as I was expecting something simple and not this traumatic. "Get yourself together Glenn."

I had to go forward from here

While I was driving home, I steadfastly resolved to accept that I had somehow ended up with cancer and that *I had to go forward from here*. This was probably one of the most important decisions I have ever made within myself.

Marilyn:

Isn't it funny how the image of a moment in time becomes etched in our memory with such odd details? This was the 'moment in time'. I can't for the life of me tell you what he was wearing but I can tell you the exact time because he was standing beside the wall oven in the kitchen which has a clock on it. Yes, 6.02pm exactly……. and my world stopped turning for what seemed like an eternity. It had been the usual frantically busy day: Glenn worked full time; I was running a wholesaling business, plus eighteen months previously we had opened a retailing business. Life had devolved into working seven days a week with long hours for both of us. We had given up the dancing we loved, most of our social life revolved around work-related functions and we had recently returned from a much needed week off on an exotic island. I walked in the door and found Glenn standing by the oven, and without approaching him for our usual 'hello hug and kiss', I stood on the other side of the kitchen bench and said: "I gather you have the results of the test?" He said: "Yes". I said: "And…?" and he answered: "I've got the big C". I have often wondered why I positioned myself with the kitchen bench between us, why I didn't go straight to him for a hug and a kiss as usual. It would be the first of many strange things I found myself doing over the next few months as things unfolded.

Anyway, needless to say, the next hour or so blurred into questions and answers about what had happened, how it had happened and the full extent of the information Glenn had to date. Needless to say, we were both in a complete state of shock and fear. As Glenn said earlier, we were both expecting a diagnosis of an ulcer, not cancer, so this had come completely out of the blue. Eventually, after finally getting-giving more than one hug and kiss! I suggested he should go and have a shower and I would put the dinner on, even though neither of us really felt like eating. At this stage, my mind was whirling, not only with a million unanswered questions but also with the practicalities of our position. You see, that's the way I cope with crisis – I go in to "practical response and organization". I'd be the one at the car accident, redirecting the traffic, mobile in hand ringing for help while also mustering whatever resources might be available – all in the same breath. Yes, you guessed it: I'm an 'organiser' – called a 'control freak' by those thinking less charitably. But certainly a useful type if you need something done, even though I might irritate you from time to time. Anyway, my priority was, not to go to pieces in front of Glenn, the last thing he needed was for me to be a blubbering mess, but I knew I just needed to scream into a pillow and s-o-o-n! The moment I heard him turn on the water, I ran to the couch, buried my head in a cushion and just howled. I was hoping the shower would cover any muffled sound and that I could 'get it out' and recover my composure before he returned.......

You see both Glenn and I both have 'forgettable' past marital experience, and at the ripe old age of 48 and 49, we found each other across a dance floor! We had had an interesting first few months – sparring with our relationship, both afraid to make a commitment due to past hurts. Eventually, we faced the fact that we both wanted the relationship, and had been totally committed to each other for about two and a half years. We both felt our relationship was everything we'd always wanted, and that we had great times (and lots of them) ahead of us, which is why we were working so damned hard to get ahead financially so we could enjoy our future together. And then this happens!

We went forward as an indivisible force
True to form, I woke up with my head full of practicalities. Like a lot of couples, we had not got around to reviewing wills etc since our time together. We didn't have powers of attorney or health directives in place, and we had never talked through the possibility of this little scenario. All of a sudden, we found ourselves facing the possibility of very few tomorrows. At that stage we did not know what was to happen on Tuesday – would the specialist advise immediate surgery and, if so, was there any risk of not surviving even that? And one thing we both needed was to know that our affairs were in order a soon as possible, so that there was one less thing to worry about, regardless of what happened next. And all of this with a background of Glenn having a twelve year old daughter on the other side of the country – fourteen hours travelling time away. Then, just when I thought "nothing can be worse than this", Glenn very quietly said: "Maybe it would be better if I move out while I get through all this because it's not fair on you". I didn't think anything could have hurt as much as the news of the original diagnosis did, but this came close. I said to him: "If I lose you to the cancer, I will survive because I will have no choice, but don't ask me to lose you by choice, that would be insufferable". We have never spoken about it since – guess we probably will though, when he reads what I have written here! Either way, the issue was settled and we went forward as an indivisible force.

Our first gift in the lining of this very dark cloud

Somehow we got through it all. By Sunday night we had a plan of action for Monday. We had asked, discussed and come up with answers to all the tough questions and the hard decisions had been made and we had found our first gift in the lining of this very dark cloud. The process of discussing the deepest, most intimate and most emotionally charged issues of our lives had strengthened what was already a very strong bond. This was now OUR fight. We were battling this wretched thing and WE were determined to win. From that time it has always been OUR cancer, not Glenn's cancer, and I think that played a very important role in his healing.

Another little gem came to light

Monday went by in a blur of meetings, phone calls, arrangement etc. AND another little gem came to light – how the universe gets behind you when you have a clearly defined purpose in mind. Somehow the whole world got behind us in what we needed to do. My first priority was to get Glenn into large doses of wheatgrass as, coincidentally, I had recently been reading about its healing qualities and lots of research had shown it had remarkable cancer killing abilities. I rang a local supplier and arranged for a juicer and trays of the growing grass to be delivered along with a kit for growing it ourselves and so we went into production. Trays and trays of grass at various stages of growth one started every two days! My next priority was to visit our local health food shop which was run by a naturopath. After she got over the shock of my news, she recommended we integrate several products into our diet, amongst them some grains and flaxseed oil. Little did I know (nor did she mention) the huge role these grains play in getting B17 into the body. By Monday night, though exhausted, we were ready for Tuesday's appointment, feeling just a little more centred. I don't know what I would have done if I had not had private health and income protection insurance. I was able to immediately take time off work on virtually my full salary and I had an insurance clause in place. At least this took away the stress of what to do about money in the near future, and gave me access to immediate treatment with top medical professionals. I found that reassuring at the time.

I had accepted the fact that I had cancer and was now going forward. However, I was still very apprehensive, on my initial visit to the surgeon, for his evaluation. The surgeon had the reputation of being one of the best around the country. My partner Marilyn was by my side. After examining all the documentation, the surgeon stated that an operation was the only cure. He said that the tumour was in the relatively early stages and I was fortunate to have it diagnosed now. He explained the process leading up to the operation and that the best results in this area were achieved by undergoing pre-surgery chemotherapy and radiation treatment. I had always had an aversion to surgery. He did instil a bit more confidence in me by the way he explained the upcoming surgery in simplistic terms. The surgeon reminded me that there were no alternatives and he had made arrangements for the next phase in this procession.

Marilyn:
From that Tuesday, within two weeks, we had visited three specialists – all with excellent reputations as the

best in their field –and had been advised to undergo chemotherapy and radiation prior to surgery. At no time was there any suggestion or advice of alternative treatment, and when each was specifically asked as to the role of nutrition, the answer was a unanimous: "Eat anything you like, just don't lose weight. Now is the time to get into hamburgers, cakes and whatever you fancy, just don't lose weight!" In a state of panic and shock, we simply accepted and agreed to go down the path of five days' chemo with fifteen treatments of radiation, started concurrently, followed by two to three weeks after the last radium. The time lag was to enable the immune system to start recovering from this horrific assault, so as to minimise the possibility of infection from surgery.

Was I still prepared to go ahead?

Another hospital, and there I was visiting more doctors referred by the surgeon. When the issue of degradation of the body's immune system was touched upon, I cringed. This really goes against all my principles as a health and safety professional. The reply that "There is no other alternative" echoes in my brain. Let's get on with it. Marilyn was by my side, as always, showing tremendous support. The waiting rooms in the main were filled with people that were generally much older and appeared as though they hadn't much time left for this world. All types of cancer were treated there. One or two patients were young people whom I felt rather sorry for, knowing what they were going through. Why them? It was a depressing place. I knew mentally I had to be strong if I was going to get through this.

The advice to eat anything was not followed, as Marilyn and I instigated a diet of healthy, nutritional juices and foods. The loss of weight didn't worry me as I knew I was eating well. Even at this stage, I knew I was going to overcome the cancer and Marilyn was there. Meditation became an important additional support during this time. I was feeling reasonably well, physically, when we met the surgeon for the final consultation before the arranged date of my operation. Mentally my mind was in a bit of turmoil. My partner (and to a lesser degree myself) had investigated the causes, effects and available treatments of cancer and we believed that there were alternatives to surgery. One of the long-term effects of removal of the oesophagus was ongoing reflux problems and, as a result, a debilitating health condition. Was I still prepared to go ahead with the operation?

Marilyn:
On the last day of radiation therapy, we had another visit from the surgeon to discuss the full details of the forthcoming surgery and what to expect post-operatively. Our discussions that first weekend led me to believe that Glenn would not be happy with the severely compromised quality of life that even the best outcome offered. However, I felt very strongly that Glenn himself had to make the decision as to whether to have the surgery or not. It was HIS life we were talking about and he really needed to be in control of the decisions we made. So I made the conscious decision to ensure he had as much information as possible before the surgery date and I started asking the surgeon some very direct questions. As we walked out of the surgery, Glenn said

that he didn't want the surgery if there were any possible alternatives. We decided to spend the three weeks we had until the surgery date to find all the information we could on cancer and its treatment. We agreed not to decide one way or the other on surgery until we had carried out further research. We left the booking for surgery in place, just in case we decided that was the best option after all.

Finally some answers
After the original diagnosis, we had already become pro-active in researching a nutritional approach, mainly on the basis of ensuring that the body was in the best possible shape to cope with the assault about to be fired at it. During our research travels, we came across a local clinic using a nutritional approach with cancer patients and they were getting encouraging results. A visit here convinced us further that surgery was in fact likely to do more harm than good, both mentally and physically. It was explained that, by ensuring we continue with a strong nutritional programme, Glenn would have every chance, not only of ridding himself of this tumour, but also warding off the development of the dreaded secondaries we had been warned about. Also, of course, without the added stress and complications of surgery, the body could use its energy and immune system to heal, rather than just survive. A week before the operation date, and after much research and discussion with many people (Marilyn was at the forefront) and many moments agonizing alone, I had made my decision. I CAN BEAT THIS WITHOUT SURGERY! Other people have done so. So can I. A great weight was lifted from my mind. I spoke to my local doctor who

expressed grave concerns about my decision. "Do you want to speak to another surgeon? There are no proven alternatives etc." I spoke to the surgeon who echoed a similar attitude of doom and gloom. We moved on.

Marilyn: *An interesting point is that, when Glenn rang to cancel surgery, the surgeon's wife asked him to keep in touch as they were very interested in our outcome. Apparently, they have another patient who opted out of surgery that is doing very well based on a nutritional approach. When we think about the fact that this approach was not mentioned in any of our visits to the doctor or surgeon, even as a support to the proposed chemo/radium/surgery recommended, it is very easy to become quite enraged. We are not in any way recommending that others should reject any form of medical recommendation. What we are saying is, that there is other information available and it can only be a benefit to be aware of all possible information before making a decision to go with any recommended treatment, whether it be medical or alternative. After all, surely a good nutritional programme can only enhance the success of any medical treatment. So the best decision may be a combination of both.*

The healing begins

The next few months involved a 'full on' implementation of nutritional support for my body in its fight against cancer. Marilyn was at times involved in researching and improving our diet. She had taken the approach that this new diet regime was a lifestyle change for both of us, not only to cure my cancer but also to enable our bodies to be in optimum health for our future years. I was very conscious of the 'radical' road we had taken and felt apprehensive on many occasions. Every tingle in my back or chest, slight difference in body function or mild spasm of indigestion was greeted with the thought that: "This is not related to that former health problem I had". It was my way of combating any negative thought. I was not going to say the word 'cancer' as my mind may take that as a direction. I wanted to be always positive about the end result. I was positive in my mind that I had overcome the most important hurdle in my life. I felt good.

Marilyn

At this point, some instinct in me told me it was time we stopped thinking of ourselves as 'recovering from cancer'. It was time to accept Glenn was free of cancer and simply think of ourselves as healthy individuals on a quest to stay that way. This mind shift was easier said than done, but we were consciously reminding ourselves that this as in fact true. I feel this was a very necessary mind-set change to make in order for us to move forward.

The time came for the first conclusive test for my being rid of the dreaded disease. Again I felt a certain amount of apprehension. It seemed consciousness returned all at once after the endoscopy. Rather anxious at the time, I asked the attending nurse when the surgeon would be visiting me. I was told he had already been and spoken to me of which, as he mentioned might happen, I didn't remember anything at all. He had left the results with his comments lying on my stomach. "Diagnosis: all clear. Congratulations". I felt immediate elation. I continued reading the rest of the words "No signs of cancer seen" with my head in the clouds. What an outcome? Where was Marilyn? I couldn't wait to tell her.

Marilyn
Eventually, Glenn emerged with a big grin. "It's gone". He said: "Gone". I said it just didn't seem real but sure enough the piece of paper in his hand said: 'normal: no signs of cancer'. Have a guess what was the one scenario we hadn't considered? This one. So, despite all our planning, we found ourselves in a state of complete and utter disbelief – albeit with a positive tone this time. In fact, we were so dazed by this wonderful result we both decided we didn't want to go home or back to the real world for a while and, instead, went to a new estate community that had grown up near our home and had a sushi lunch and spent the afternoon looking at display homes! I think it took a good week for the news to really sink in and for us to come back to earth. One of the horrid side effects of a life threatening diagnosis is that it is always at the back of the mind. Every time I have some discomfort, or indigestion it raises the spectre of: "Is it back?" and both Marilyn and I know we had to reject that thought and concentrate on all the indicators that this phase in our lives has now passed and that I am well.

The future beckons both myself and Marilyn
I feel comfortable that, even though my immune system is still below par, it will eventually return to normal. I am well and will continue to feel well and the future beckons both me and Marilyn.

A little advice

Our aim in sharing our experiences with you was, firstly, to underline that our bodies are capable of beating even the diseases our medics deem to be incurable, without THEIR intervention.

Secondly, to let you know what we did, so that you have some immediate practical course of action to start on while you do your own research. Each of us has to take responsibility for our own health and well-being, rather than leaving it in the hands and minds of others.

Consequently, we suggest that you seek out books and websites yourself, by simply asking around or typing in your particular health concern into your web browser. You will be amazed at the enormous quantity of information that is freely available, and how often 'just the right book' falls into your lap. We encourage you to read and research for yourself until, like us, you become convinced that you or your loved one can improve your health by aiding your body to function at its best. We hope that somewhere amongst our stories, you will find the inspiration and/or information you need to create your own 'wellness miracle'.

Centre of Living Hope

I have deliberately set this two page chapter in the centre of my book between Thrivers' inspiring stories. This is the heart of 'Flying Free' and the heart of each Thriver's story reflecting the limitless power that is at the core of each one of us. Unfortunately we do not always realise this until we have a crisis in our lives, but the wonderful thing is that it is there, always.

Be still
and you will
feel me.

Listen
and you will
hear me.

Look
and you will
See.

Know
I am here
Always.

Centre of Living Hope

We are all one united by all that is loving, no matter who we are, where we are, what we do, what we have or have not. We are one. As one we radiate. Hope is the light of the spirit. Hope transforms everything it touches into glorious light and endless possibilities. Hope shines. Hope cleanses, opens, renews, beautifies, inspires, and heals. We need water and air to survive; we need hope to thrive. Hope is free and so are we!

'but those who hope in the LORD will renew their strength; they will fly up on wings like eagles.
They will run and not be tired; they will walk and not be weary'.

Isaiah 40:31

'Let us have endless hope, limitless
love and complete faith
In the wonder of God within us
to heal beyond ourselves
and bathe in glorious, divine light
We are truly blessed!'

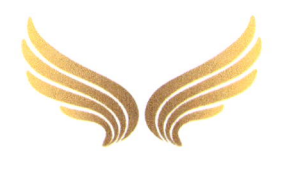

"My life so far had provided enough stressful experiences for ten lifetimes, as previously mentioned. But gradually, one by one, I made peace with them all"

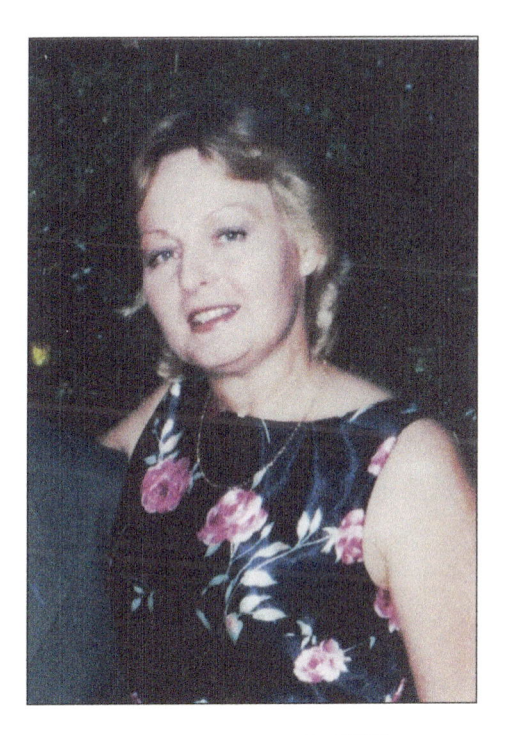

MARILYN BENNETT

I met Marilyn as a patient at The Oasis of Hope Hospital in Tijuana, Mexico in 2008. I was struck by her exuberance and grasp of life. I connected with her energy and powerful attitude. She was amazing and fully immersed and committed to her treatment: wonderful and at the same time, rare to see. Marilyn shares her feisty, determined, uplifting healing in her own written words with Glenn, her partner (in previous chapter) by her side. The strength they were for each other shines through the challenging times.

Here Marilyn shares her feisty, determined story with you to share with you:

My name is Marilyn Bennett and I am based in Brisbane, Australia.

I turn 60 today, 13 Feb 2013! I am married, with 4 adult children and ten grandchildren aged from nineteen down to two. The kids tell me there will be no more "kid's kids!" I would describe myself as a spiritualist, believing in a benevolent, totally fair energy I refer to as Source, rather than following any particular faith or creed, but I certainly believe in Christian principles when it comes to my value base. I have been the Chief Executive Officer of my own company, a snack-food wholesaler, since 1991, although these days I am semi-retired and the company is now mainly run by my children.

My priorities in life prior to diagnosis were, if asked, my husband, family and then work, but in reality when I look back it was inevitably a case of "hubby and the kids can wait and this work matter needs my urgent attention." So while I would never hesitate to give my time to them if they asked or had an urgent need, I cannot honestly say they held prior place for my attention. You may also notice that there is no mention of time for ME in the list at all! In fact most people who know me will tell you their summation of me would have been "workaholic", and I would have to agree with them. But more of that later.

Prior to diagnosis, there were many other stresses in my life. My Dad had recently died and I was not ready for him to go, and was working hard enough to avoid the grieving. I was juggling a second business, an online business and investment properties with renovations and tenants thrown in. I also managed our superannuation fund! Keeping up with changing legislation for tenants, tax and super funds is almost a full time job in itself, let alone the administration of these functions.

Needless to say, I was also overweight and very unfit, due to a lot of travelling and time spent away from home in motels and eating out. Looking back, I never "made" time for myself at all – not even to exercise or eat well, and overall, compared to where I am now, I would describe my pre-cancer life as highly stressed, very driven and overall very unsatisfying, even though I have always enjoyed most aspects of my role.

Diagnosed at the age of 55 with a tumour on my right ovary

I was diagnosed in 2008 at the age of 55 with a tumour on my right ovary. It was an early diagnosis due to an odd circumstance. You see, in 2003, my husband Glenn had been diagnosed with oesophageal cancer and, after some initial 'pre-surgery chemo and radiation', elected not to have the barbaric surgery recommended as 'his only course of action'. On top of running the two businesses and everything else, I spent all my 'spare' time researching for alternative solutions and putting together an alternative programme based on stress reduction, organic eating and naturopathic support. This resulted in his being totally clear of the cancer in 11 months, which is basically unheard of. You will now have read his story in the previous chapter.

As a result of this experience, I had added a cancer marker to my annual health checks and, lo and behold, it came back with a high reading in 2008. But two factors were different for me. Firstly, I had seen the effects of a 'cleaner' lifestyle in Glenn's recovery and, secondly, while he had been able to simply take 6 months off from work to recover, I headed a company that was not structured so that I could simply walk away for six months as he did. Consequently, I made the decision that, as it was a very early diagnosis, I would take some time to get my company and staff to a stage where they could cope without me while I recovered (as Glenn had done) and in the meantime do my best to incorporate some lifestyle changes, particularly in relation to nutrition. The plan was to take three months off in 2009, go overseas, completely away from the business, and recover.

Looking back, I now notice two things – just how much of a priority my work was, which horrifies me, and secondly, just how much faith I had that I would recover, which is probably the main thing that finally got me through! Problem was, as I have learned, Source becomes impatient when I decide to delay getting my priorities in order, and in April 2009 my eldest nephew came home from a gym session, sat down, drank a glass of water and didn't get up again. The autopsy showed he had blown his aorta (major blood vessel to the heart) out and nothing would have saved him. This boy was the eldest child of my beloved baby sister (and only sibling: we have no brothers) and big sisters are supposed to be able to help and protect baby sisters and of course there wasn't a damned thing I could do to even make this better, let alone fix it.

The stress took me from single tumour/under control to Stage 4 metastasized (with a second tumour and cancer throughout my abdomen) inoperable, ovarian cancer in 6 weeks! "Your job as the patient, and ours as Doctors, is to give your body the right support to enable it to do what it is designed to do – heal!" The Oasis of Hope Hospital in Playas, Mexico (just over the border from San Diego) had been our Plan B if the regime we worked out for Glenn had not worked. Consequently, I contacted them and, after sending my tests over, they rang me, discussed my options and advised me to get over there a.s.a.p.

On arrival, one of the first things I was told was: "We can't cure your cancer" which was the last thing I wanted to hear, having flown literally half way round the world, travelling some 36 hours to be treated. However, they went on to say something that became a very powerful basis for my recovery: "Your body will do the healing, your job as the patient, and ours as Doctors, is to give your body the right support to enable it to do what it is designed to do – heal!" At this point it got my attention! The second thing I didn't want to hear was a recommendation for chemotherapy! I had spent nearly 6 years running a website we put up after Glenn's experience, promoting the benefits and power of diet and lifestyle, and when I had initially researched The Oasis of Hope Hospital they were only using natural therapies. However, they explained that in 2005 they incorporated chemotherapy into their regimes and were getting 15% better survival results with this protocol. They also explained that the other therapies they incorporated would protect my body from the full-on ravages of chemo and also make the cancer more receptive to the chemo and therefore I should need less treatments overall. I decided to go with their recommendation, although it took a lot of tears and counselling by their emotional support team for me to get to a place where I could accept the chemo as my friend.

It turned out to be an excellent decision, as, after just the second round of treatment (incorporating the chemo), I was in remission. The second tumour and all the spots of cancer in my abdomen had disappeared and the primary tumour had shrunk from grapefruit size back down to the size of a wine cork. It was also calcified! When I had a scan back in Australia, the pathologist described it as "the possible residuum from a previously described ovarian tumour". My interpretation of that is that he had never seen anything like it before and didn't quite know what to make of it. Then I was given four possible scenarios. I could have the 'residuum' removed, however, was warned that any surgery could, in fact, result in a spread of cancer, particularly as my immune system had taken the hit of two chemo treatments, or we could leave it there and one of two things would happen. Either it would stay there and never bother me again, or it might even disappear as my body 'cleaned it up' once my immune system recovered. The fourth scenario was that it might reactivate. When I asked what we would do if it reactivated the reply was: "Repeat what we've done, but if it does reactivate we will have to get it out." As I had two chances out of three that I wouldn't have to have any more treatment or surgery, I opted to let it sit.

I resumed my life, but with a lot of alterations

So I resumed my life, but with a lot of alterations. I spent a lot of time reflecting who I was, what I wanted, and what I had lived so far in this life. I made peace with a childhood with emotionally unavailable alcoholic parents, sexual abuse by a teacher, betrayal by more than one husband/partner, a case of incest, years of single motherhood/breadwinner, including a bankruptcy due to going into business with a 'friend', and the death of a father I had learned to love late in life, and only just started to really know, and, of course, the death of my beloved nephew.

I developed a very strong faith in Source, and a very solid and supportive understanding of how life works. I cut down on work commitments and spent much more time with family, friends and on things I wanted to be doing. We also bought a large fifth wheeler (like a horse float but with living space) and put tenants in our home. I handed over management of our properties to property managers and Glenn and I started a much more leisurely lifestyle.

Now, remember I said earlier that Source has a way of becoming 'impatient' when we continue to ignore the hints we are given along the way that we are out of balance? Well, as much as I had made some major, major changes to every aspect of my life and attitude, and was thoroughly convinced that I was no longer suffering from any real stress, it seems Source's scorecard did not match mine. Consequently, after just over two years in remission, the 'residuum' started to reactivate. Its timing was abysmal, as we were about to embark on

3 months overseas, but, based on the good response we had had in 2009, we made a decision (with my Doctor's approval) to delay treatment until after our trip. Problem was my 'little friend' made the most of being given some extra 'play time'. By the time we returned from our travels in November 2011, my markers were sky high again and, although I had no metastases, the tumour was growing rapidly.

I was still taking responsibility for the welfare of everyone associated with my company

At this point, I 'lost it', big time! I looked back over the past couple of years of remission and reviewed where I thought I was at. I felt I had reduced my stress levels enormously – a factor I thought was an absolute key to good health – and I had certainly improved my overall lifestyle and my diet, and I certainly had plans for the future that I was enthusiastic about. Overall, I felt I was in the best place I had ever been in my life! Because of this, I lost my confidence in my ability to recover from this second onslaught. I just couldn't see my way through it. After all I had done and was doing, all the things I was so convinced were the keys to recovery and a long happy and healthy life, but now had evidence (by the reactivation of the cancer) that, in fact, the very foundation that I built my life on, was incorrect. My confidence was shaken to the core because I was thinking that everything I believed in had been shattered.

Fortunately I have a son who has a very similar outlook on life to mine. I am convinced we reincarnated this time in order to be each other's guiding light in all matters spiritual, as we have come to understand life, almost hand in hand. So much so, that I was able to unload my darkest thoughts and feelings, including that I thought perhaps it was just 'my time to go' and that I wasn't feeling any desire to fight any more. His answer was a very calm: "well Mum, if that is what you really feel, then you will get no argument from me and I'll support you all I can". This in itself is huge, because I have also had a lot of experiences with this son to know that he loves me deeply and that the last thing he wants personally is for me to pass over any time soon!

However, he went on to ask: "What makes you think everything you believe is wrong?" I replied: "because I have done everything I know how to do. And overall I have been feeling so much more at peace and so much less stressed than I have ever been and still the cancer has returned." He said: "Well, I agree with you that you have made enormous changes over the past couple of years, and I have been blown away with the depth of insight you have developed and some of the enlightened thoughts you have shared with me. I have also seen a huge difference in the way you interact with the family, but Mum, I gotta tell you, when it comes to work, you are every bit as stressed as you always were." I knew he had scored a bullseye, as I felt a firm 'thud' in my solar plexus. As we discussed things further, I realised that I had come to understand that everyone of us comes into this life and lives our own experience. I had come to know that everyone whose actions or lack of actions in the past had caused me to feel hurt in anyway, had behaved the way they had out of the pain of their own experience or their own lack of feeling loved, worthy and balanced. I had released all my expectations of others, given up my role of 'Miss Responsible for everyone and everything', stopped bleeding whenever I saw someone else 'doing it the hard way', and relaxed into the understanding that everyone, including myself, was in the perfect place at the perfect time, having the perfect experience to move them forward to a better experience. This understanding had given me a peace that I had never experienced before.

BUT I had not applied this understanding to my business life. I was still taking responsibility for the welfare of everyone associated with my company, including staff and distributors. If a distributor didn't make a success of their business, I felt responsible, even though I had offered help that they had refused! And the thought that my company might fold, putting my staff out of work and my distributors out of business was unthinkable, even if it ended up being because I had cancer or even died!!!! Once I applied the same philosophy to my business relationships as I did to my personal ones, things became so much clearer. After all, I hadn't held a gun to anyone's head to join my staff or become a distributor for my business. In fact they were fortunate to be given the opportunity as, unlike a lot of business owners, I had always and would always, do my very best to give them the best possible support while associated with my company. What they did with that opportunity was up to them, and I owed them nothing more than respect in my ongoing relationship with them. Once I came to terms with the fact that I was not personally responsible for their welfare, I had an enormous feeling of relief, as though the weight of the world had been lifted off my shoulders. I had absolutely no clue, before my son's comment, of the huge amount of stress I had still been carrying, stress made even worse by my perceived inability to spend as much time as I used to working in the business. I finally understood that stress reduction was not achieved by avoiding a situation (or minimising contact with it) but by changing one's attitude to that situation so that I no longer experienced stress in my association with it. Furthermore, I understood why the cancer had reactivated. Once again it came back bearing gifts – and the first gift was the life changing insight I had just experienced. Once again I felt empowered to move forward with my treatments and a knowing that I was right on track.

Unfortunately my little 'friend' was still causing more havoc

Due to the very quick and effective response I had to the two chemo treatments in 2009, I thought that perhaps we could get enough reduction of the tumour to make it safely operable by just using the Vitamin C protocols, something my Doctors agreed was worth a try. Sure enough, we got a nice big reduction in the size of the tumour after the first treatment, and so we agreed on a second Vitamin C treatment four weeks later. Unfortunately, almost immediately after the second Vitamin C treatment, I fell ill with a strain of 'flu that was putting my fellow Aussies in bed and/or in hospital for up to three weeks, and after having tests done prior to what was to be my third Vitamin C treatment, we found the tumour had started its rampage again. So, the decision was made to go straight back on to a chemo regime, followed by further surgery in June 2012! Unfortunately, my little 'friend' was still causing more havoc than we realised, so my poor surgeon found himself dealing with several complications that took him and his team six and a half hours to sort out.

On waking up in ICU the following morning, I found I couldn't move my left leg. This caused quite a hilarious situation because my surgeon had asked the nursing staff to keep an eye on my right leg as he had had to scrape the muscle to get the best margins on the tumour and was concerned he may have damaged its function. So when I said I couldn't feel or move my left leg there was great confusion. This was rectified later by my very patient physios who managed to keep me safe while I forced the other muscles in my thigh to support me and give me enough movement to be able to walk with the aid of a walker, and to go up and down stairs, albeit one foot at a time and with both hands on the rails.

I was then scheduled to have another three rounds of chemotherapy, but in Australia. My Oasis Doctors assured me that, having had the supportive alternative therapy back-up treatments, my body had been primed and, through taking the home supplements, I would be OK to have the chemo in Australia. This was great news on several fronts. Firstly, no cost for treatments or travel, and, secondly, no stresses of travelling half way round the world for treatments. However, without the support of the supplements, my body just could not handle the onslaught of the chemo treatments, and I bounced between unacceptably low immune function tests and urinary tract infections. After weeks of further surgeries, ducking and diving with more chemo sessions and later radiation, completing on January 11th 2012, the good news was that I was finally declared 'in remission' and cancer free! I am pleased to say, I came through the experience very well, with minimal side effects. I think a combination of positive attitude, good diet and supplementation when I could manage it throughout the whole treatment process, were all factors in my getting through so much better than many others I met and observed throughout my dance with cancer.

I had an interesting chat with one of the drivers who took me into my treatments, and he said that he had found that patients who had taken an active role in their cancer treatment and had added natural therapy support to their regime seemed to do a lot better than those who relied solely on the treatments offered by their Doctors and the hospitals. My surgeon also, very openly, credits my recovery largely to the alternative treatments I undertook. He has told me, more than once, that when he diagnosed me as 'inoperable', his thoughts were: "Oh no, this is another one I am going to lose!" He puts my recovery down to a combination of the choices I made regarding my treatment and my determination to be healed. In fact he said to me just before my radiation "that 'cure' is not a word we usually use with cancer, but provided you have the radiation treatments, I think I can say that you will have the cure you told me you were looking for when you first came to me."

We have far more control over our health than we ever thought possible!

Needless to say, now that both my husband Glenn and I have recovered from cancers that were deemed to be almost certainly unbeatable, I am often asked to what

I credit our respective recoveries. The interesting thing is I think both our recoveries were due to the same factors:

1. An attitude of "This is not a death sentence, just something that needs to be worked through, and my body's way of letting me know I need to make some SERIOUS changes."
2. A radical and immediate programme of stress reduction
3. A radical and immediate diet change
4. A radical and immediate re-evaluation of what was important in our lives and what we wanted going forward

So having been asked to share our approach with you, here goes: "We have far more control over our health than we ever thought possible!" Glenn's mantra was: "The medics don't have a clue as to how to beat the common cold, but my body handles that OK, so this is just another thing my body can heal." My view was: "As I have witnessed the positives in our lives from Glenn's experience, there have to be some gifts in this too".

We had become very aware that stress was the biggest factor in all dis-ease, a factor that is now scientifically documented in a book called Biology of Belief by Bruce Lipton. Bruce is a medically qualified cellular biologist who has proved, through scientifically documented experiments in petri dishes, that our thinking processes produce chemical reactions in our bodies that either damage or nurture our cells. This leaves no doubt that we have far more control over our health than our societal conditioning would have us believe we do. That in itself is one of the most empowering pieces of information I have become aware of during my dance with cancer and in itself a huge gift! So began a soul searching journey, particularly for myself, as to what issues I was thinking about in a way that was causing me to create harmful stress chemicals, rather than allowing my body to get on with being the naturally inclined healing mechanism it was designed to be. And, boy! Did I have fertile ground to search!

My life so far had provided enough stressful experiences for ten lifetimes, as previously mentioned. But gradually, one by one, I made peace with them all.

What hope has the body got of healing, if we simply pour the 'poisonous hormones of stress' in on top of the good stuff! This was achieved through the 'change of perspective' that came about through, firstly, understanding the physical implications of stress (as per Dr Lipton's research) and, secondly, through an acceptance that I was not responsible for anyone else's outcomes other than my own. This insight was further reinforced by realising that this was exactly what Glenn had had to come to terms with, and what every cancer survivor I had met had come to terms with.

I had an interesting experience following one of my overseas' treatments. At lunch one day there were seven of us around the table. When I spoke to Glenn that night, I told him I thought I would be the only one still alive within 6 months, and, sadly, I was. What had given me that insight? Simply listening to the conversation! Each of my fellow diners were still locked into the stress caused by believing that they were the victims of other people and situations, and none had done a single thing about changing their attitude towards anything that was causing them stress. Yes, they were all religiously taking their medications and abiding by the recommended diet – but what hope has the body got of healing if we simply pour in the 'poisonous hormones of stress' on top of the good stuff.

This convinced us both, even more, of the key importance of stress reduction in recovery, and we came to understand that this could be achieved simply by changing one's perspective of whatever/whoever was the trigger for the stress. We came to see that 'stress', like 'beauty', is 'all in the eye of the beholder'. Of course, changing one's perspective on life can, like everything else, be viewed as difficult or even impossible, but if we can just 'live with the possibility' that there may be a better way to view things, and continually ask: "How could there be some good/benefit in this situation?" then, invariably, our inner wisdom will aid us by giving us a better perspective. It does take effort, initially, as we are so programmed to respond (knee-jerk like) to everything we experience, but in a surprisingly short time, you will find yourself automatically looking for the advantage or gift in every situation.

For Glenn and I the gift was life!

A little advice

If I were asked to sum up our approach, it would be: re-evaluate and question everything – your understanding of life, any treatment advice given to you, your diet, lifestyle, family, work, recreation time – looking specifically for stressing/unhelpful factors, and change/improve things wherever possible, because the very act of taking control, even over little things, empowers you energetically, to say nothing of changing your body chemistry in ways that allow your body to heal – and last but not least, look for the gift in EVERYTHING!

"I always knew there was so much more!"

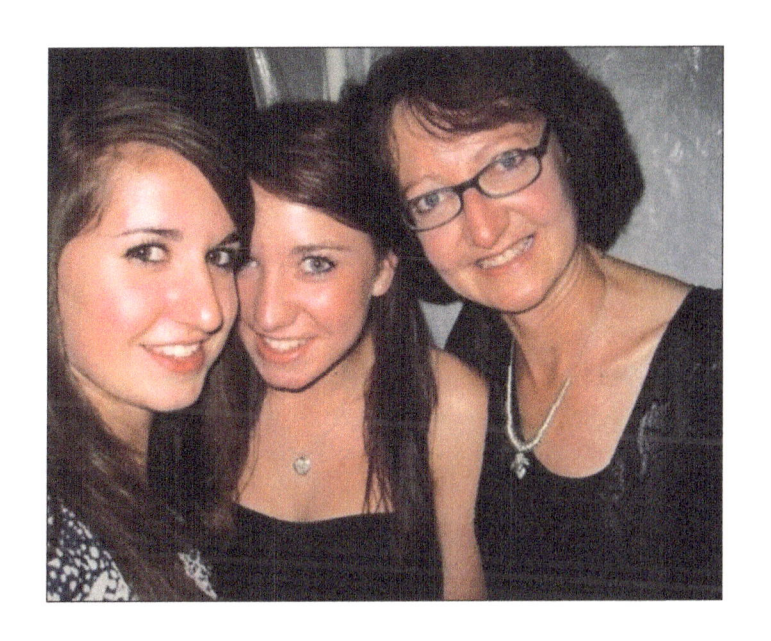

HELEN MORGAN

Helen and I met briefly once at a Breast Friends' support group meeting one evening in Aylesbury. Six months later, my healing story: 'Hidden Gifts' was published and Helen called me out of the blue. I remembered her from what she said before: "I am on chemo, I wonder if it's working!" And she remembered my talking about 'Post-mastectomy Sex' a chapter from my book at that same meeting. What was I thinking!

Later, when she chose to resign from her job and take time out, I asked her a few weeks later, if she was missing working, having worked all her life. Her spontaneous reply said it all: "I always knew there was so much more!" Here her beautiful daughters Laura and Sabrina tell their story:

Climbing a sheer mountain!

There's so much to say about Mum's love of Yosemite National Park and why a beautiful landscape picture of it was hanging on her bedroom wall for as long as we could remember. She found it magical and enchanting, in awe of its nature; it was her place of fascination, and the dream to aim for.

Mum was never afraid of a challenge, and once she had her mind set on something, she followed it through until she'd achieved her goal. 2003 was the year she was able to take forward her challenge of climbing Half Dome Mountain in Yosemite, and she spent months training for it beforehand. For us, being just 13 and 10 at the time, school took priority and we didn't go to America with her – after all, we were much too young to go climbing a sheer mountain! However we do remember her going for daily walks and hikes with a rucksack full of rocks and a bottle of water. At this point we had no idea of the enormity of her challenge.

When it came round to the day of her climb, she was nervous, but confident her training would pay off. She was right, and made it easily through each of the checkpoints en route, up to the base of the very peak where the last part of the climb was up an almost vertical rock face. After all this expense of energy and determination, the last thing you want to see when you get this far is a thunderstorm brewing overhead. As the storm continued to worsen and get closer, there was a risk of lightning striking the metal structure to which she was harnessed, leaving her waiting on a mountainside in the hope that it would pass by. She had enough energy left to continue to the top, but an instructor eventually told her it was too dangerous to carry on or stay put, forcing her to retreat back to the log cabin. Although we are not sure how long she waited, we know she stuck it out for as long as she could because she hated to be defeated by something as petty as the weather. It must have been so disheartening for her, but, none the less, we remember her coming back joyous and excited about her trip and adventure.

Yosemite was Mum's favourite place and it formed the background for her love of travel and exploration. This then continued into our family holidays, which are where some of our fondest memories of our time together lie. Going away with Mum was all about exploring, immersing ourselves in a new culture, and having an adventure. Mum had not only travelled abroad but lived abroad too, in Malaya, Singapore and Libya, then later in the USA before returning home to have us. We always questioned why she gave up her annual pass to Disneyland California to come back to rainy England! Her love for travel and exploration was passed onto both of us as we are always eager to travel and experience new places.

We knew what we had to do

Even though we were a tight-knit little family of three, we thought it was important to write this section separately, from our own perspectives, as we remember different aspects and experienced different emotions.

Sabrina:

I remember when I was first told that Mum had breast cancer. I was in my room dancing around as I usually was, when she asked me to sit on the bed as she had some news she needed to tell me. Naturally, she was upset and started crying, and at the age of 14 I took it upon myself to comfort her and tell her not to worry, because she would always have Laura and myself by her side for love and support. I realised very quickly that Laura and I needed to be the mature daughters she had brought us up to be.

I don't recall talking to Laura about it after as we were told separately, but as we appear to be mystically connected by thoughts (no, we're not twins, but a lot of people are surprised when we tell them there's a three year age gap!), we knew what we had to do and we made the best of a bad situation.

Laura:

I remember being in the kitchen, sat at the table, when Mum came in through the front door completely unable to hide the fact that she was trying to hide something. It felt like an eternity before she told me what had happened, whilst every tragedy apart from cancer whirled through my head. She eventually told me that she had found a lump in her breast, that the doctors said it was cancer, and that she would need an operation to remove the tumour.

It then took another lifetime for that to sink in, before I could get my head around how to respond. I told her how comforting it was that they'd caught it early, that they could remove it easily, and that chemotherapy would cure it completely. I felt strongly that a positive

Sabrina:
When Mum had her first operation, I was on a school cruise to Egypt. Possibly one of the hardest and strangest situations to be in... Mum's going in for a major operation and I'm sailing away to another country! The school had told us that we weren't allowed to take our mobile phones on the trip, but, due to the circumstances, I was the only pupil who was allowed to take mine.

Thankfully, I didn't receive any emergency calls, only texts from Laura and Mum to tell me everything went well and she was recovering quickly. I thoroughly enjoyed the trip, despite what was going on at home and came back with many stories and photographs to share with her to cheer her up.

Laura:
Biology class – what a fitting lesson to be stuck in whilst your mother is having an operation... Well, the solution here is to cry, be rude to the teacher, and storm out of class to go and sit in the loos all lesson, all without explaining to the teacher what is wrong... In hindsight, this didn't really help me or the teacher, but I sure would not have learnt anything in that class!

When Mum came home from the hospital I remember being astounded at how able she was, considering she'd just had a breast removed. She didn't complain, moan or say she was in pain – that was one of Mum's best traits, being strong and carrying on.

The energy and determination was phenomenal

What a fantastic help support groups are, especially those witty enough to joke about the one condition that all members share. 'Breast Friends' is a support group in Aylesbury and surrounding areas for anyone diagnosed with breast cancer. It was there that Mum met Jacinta, who soon became her 'soul sister' and cherished friend – the author of this book. Mum met so many people at Breast Friends, and they would get together for regular coffees, dinners and more coffees!

She was thankful to have met and gained the friendship of all these people who were going through the same life changing experience as her, and who provided her with a great deal of the support that someone with cancer needs. Although having family around you when going through a difficult time is important, it can be friends that people often feel more able to open up to. For Mum, having this extra group of friends was priceless; being able to share both the good times and the bad with people who were going through the same health worries as she was meant such a lot to her. Together, Breast Friends decided to sign up for the Relay for Life, which took place at Aylesbury Rugby club one summer weekend. Relay for Life is Cancer Research UK's annual fundraising event, where teams get together to continuously carry a baton round a track for 24 hours solid. It invites people to come together and take part in a community event that involves working as a team, aiming for a target, and raising money for Cancer Research UK.

Gladly, we volunteered to join the team and help with the task of 'relaying' continuously for 24 hours. There was such a huge mix of people taking part in the overall event, from young children to teenagers around our age, and the elderly. After doing our laps and passing the baton on to another team member, Mum told us to go home and get some proper sleep before coming back the next day, instead of camping with her in the back of the car. (We were rather disappointed at this, but then it meant we were able to do another stint the next day, before the 24 hours was up).

If you're thinking of doing a charity event, this is the one to do. We've both done the Race for Life, which is enjoyable as an individual achievement, but there is something so much more rewarding and fulfilling about the Relay. What's best is that you can choose your own team of people, which makes the relay and camping out extra special. Despite being the youngest and only people on our team that had never been diagnosed with cancer, we looked the most tired – no-one else seemed outwardly knackered after being awake and walking for so long. We couldn't understand it! The energy and determination within the Breast Friends' group was phenomenal, and you could tell it meant so much to each person.

One person who has dedicated her time and ambitions to cancer awareness is Mum's all time heroine – Ellen MacArthur. Although we did not go with her, we both remember how excited Mum was to meet Ellen MacArthur at a breakfast fundraiser for the Ellen MacArthur Cancer Trust in 2011. It was a fundraiser challenge, involving supporters climbing the 843 steps to the top of the BT tower in London, where they were greeted with breakfast and a talk from Ellen. Mum came back with a certificate and such pride to have met Ellen and been a part of her fundraiser event.

Mum was really inspired by Ellen's achievement of sailing solo around the world in 2005, and was obsessed with tracking her progress online. We remember it being as important to her as watching the 6 o'clock news – a quick check to see where Ellen had made it to that day. Mum was totally inspired by her phenomenal sailing achievement and dedication to childhood cancer awareness, perhaps sparking Mum's desire to also provide such important messages to others.

Yes, Yes, Yes I would love to. Wow!

It was during this period of her life that Mum really learnt not to let her rosy cheeks prevent her from doing something she was passionate about. The three of us have really rosy cheeks, made worse when having to do public speaking. But Mum learnt to accept and even embrace it, using the nickname 'Rosy Cheeks' to refer to herself. She had always been keen to write a book. Signing it off under a different name was exciting to her, as no one would know who wrote it.

In the end, instead of writing her messages down, she would speak them aloud. It seemed as though Mum grew out of her public speaking phobia as her cancer treatment and recovery continued. The support that she received from friends, Breast Friends and family gave her the confidence to deliver two cancer awareness presentations to schools.

My Comment as Author and Helen's spiritual buddy:
I remember Helen sitting chatting in my front room one morning, excitedly and hesitantly mentioning that she would like to speak to schools about cancer but would need training on how to do it. At that very moment, her phone rang. It was the Head of Sabrina's school ringing to ask her if she would be free to talk later that same week! She looked at me with both wonder and dread, asking me: "What shall I do?" To which I excitedly replied: "What do you want to do?" Back on the phone her wonder took over: "Yes, yes, yes, I would love to." Wow! And she had never done it before. I am so glad we were together to celebrate.

Instead of viewing cancer simply as a negative, she realised that, actually, she could use her own experience to educate young women about the signs and symptoms of breast cancer, helping women to realise a diagnosis as early as possible. Having spent hours researching and putting together a presentation, Mum went into our high school and delivered an inspirational talk to the year group above Sabrina. Unfortunately, Sabrina was not allowed to attend the speech but was beaming inside and out when she overheard girls talking in the common room about how inspiring and interesting this mysterious woman named Helen was. Mum also gave her talk to Wycombe High School where we are sure her message was equally as memorable for the girls there.

'The alien' was what Mum called it

Two years later, another bombshell... Mum was diagnosed with bowel cancer. A tumour the size of a small orange had grown in her bowel, causing her excruciating pain as it blocked her system. For both of us, this was a massive shock, as Mum seemed to have made a full recovery after breast cancer, chemotherapy, herceptin and radiotherapy.

The scary thing was that it was completely unrelated to the breast cancer and had been growing for an unknown number of years. Bowel cancer was something that we knew even less about, so we took it upon ourselves to be much more involved this time, making sure she was explaining everything to us as she went to see various doctors and specialists. Being slightly older this time, it helped us to engage more and realise the impact bowel cancer can have upon someone's life.

Mum was as brave as ever and still continued her day-to-day life as best she could without complaining or batting an eyelid at the news. However, the operation to remove the tumour this time also involved the removal of a large extent of Mum's bowel, resulting in her having to have a stoma bag fitted. Mum's bowel now exited on her midriff, covered by a small, concealed pouch. Being very squeamish, we didn't expect to find the concept so interesting to talk about. For a while we were in too much confusion or embarrassment to take a proper look at the result of the surgery. But after a few days we both assisted as best we could when she had to change the bag, and there were many times when we found ourselves sat amazed at how her bowel now worked. The part of her bowel that was visible on her midriff was moving and contracting just as it does inside everyone, amazing to watch from an outside perspective.

HELEN

'The alien' was what Mum called it. We secretly imagine she was just as fascinated as us! This was another period of Mum's life where most people would be horrified and upset by what had happened to her, but she embraced it and didn't let it get her down.

It was during this time that Mum started to take morphine for the pain she was in, as a result of the cancer, the chemotherapy and the operation. Having regular doses of morphine caused Mum to come out with some hilarious statements. Our personal favourite morphine story was a time that both of us were sat by her bedside and she asked Laura to pass her a glass of water. After staring at it for a long while, she looked up with a completely blank expression and said: "No I don't want it, there are little men peeing in here!" We could not contain ourselves and literally burst out laughing! Mum then joined in too after we explained to her what she had just said! Laughing so much that it turns into tears of happiness really is the best medicine, and a good muscle work out too! Having realised what she said was completely ridiculous, she decided to drink her water as if nothing had happened before, erupting with laughter once more.

A few days after Laura's 21st birthday, we found out that the doctors had classed Mum's condition as terminal, and she spent some time in and out of Florence Nightingale Hospice in Stoke Mandeville. The hospice cannot be thanked enough for all the love and attention they paid to our mother. During her time there, we became quite good friends with some of the nurses as they equally looked after us, and were forever telling us how amazing our Mum was. Many of the nurses said she was their favourite patient due to her happy, upbeat attitude and her constant smile. She had a knack of making everyone around her feel happy even though the surroundings were saying otherwise.

Mum's cancer diagnoses brought the three of us closer together. We had always been a tight-knit little family, but such a life changing experience for all of us meant we shared the highs and the lows, the laughter and the crying and became even more of a trio during those last few months.

Christmas 2011 was the best we had ever had

The moral of this section is that you CAN carry on, and it is NOT wrong to want to do this, although cliché, "your mother wouldn't want to see you in this state would she?" is such an important saying to us now.

Christmas 2011 was the best Christmas we had ever had, despite the circumstances. For a change, we had the family over to ours instead of going to our grandparents' house, which made for a different and exciting Christmas. Mum really appreciated having all her close family around her during the special festive season, and especially enjoyed having others cook us Christmas lunch! We had beautiful food, lots of games and laughter. Even though Mum went to bed during the day, due to being so tired, she told us afterwards that lying in bed and listening to the rest of the family laughing together made her smile inside and out. Christmas that year really made us appreciate the value of family and it helped everyone connect just that bit more. There were no showing signs of the knowledge it was Mum's last

Christmas, and it was a perfect celebration of our 'Fox' family, three weeks before Mum passed away. She passed away at the Florence Nightingale Hospice in Stoke Mandeville, a graceful sanctuary for people with life-limiting illness, and a charity we will always support. Hospices are 'ironically' a lifeline for people and their families, putting some personality into a healthcare place, rather than a clinical hospital. It certainly does help a person and their family and friends to connect more positively in such surroundings. It's when you get home that it hits you, and this is not the time for A-level exams or university dissertations to be set...

Sabrina's story:
Mum passed away at the end of January, and I had an A-level exam 4 days later. Of course my initial reaction was to push the thought out of my head and not even contemplate taking it. However, after some more thought, I encouraged myself to sit the exam, and surprisingly it turned out to be my best grade!

Living by myself and having to revise for the rest of my A-level exams proved difficult, as I had no one to motivate me. Revising was dull and I lacked my usual enthusiasm, especially as Laura was at university most of the time. However, later that year I found out that I had gained a place at the University of Brighton which was my first choice. I was absolutely over the moon and I knew I had made Mum proud.

The summer before I started university I ran the Race for Life with one of my close friends. We dedicated the run to Mum and managed to raise a substantial amount of money. I'm not one for running, or sport in general for that matter, so even though it was a fairly short run it was a struggle. I kept telling myself, you're doing this to raise money for charity to help people who are suffering with cancer. Stop being so pathetic and RUN! I managed to finish the 3 mile run in around 40 minutes, not a great time but at least I finished, despite the near on monsoon that was happening at the time. It was an emotional, yet very fun day, and I would highly recommend this to anyone!

That whole year was extremely tough, but as soon as September came around I knew the hard work and persistence had paid off. My first two years of university have been absolutely amazing and I'm so glad I put in the work that I did. I have been continuing my motivated work ethic and due to this I am now completing my Industrial Placement year at Canon UK Ltd.

Laura's story:
After a good while at home (I have absolutely no idea how many weeks it was) with Sabrina and our grandparents, I made the difficult decision to go back to university. I decided to continue with my final year of study, rather than deferring until the next year, and I have never been more focused on my academic work throughout my whole education. I breezed through my dissertations, loving every minute of researching and writing on topics close to my heart. I was awarded my first 'firsts' for my two dissertations – the only two pieces of work I did after Mum passed away.

Although I continued to regret going back to university throughout this time, and for some time afterwards, I know Mum would say I made the right choice. My grades also showed I was capable of carrying on, and I graduated with an upper second class degree that same summer.

Right after graduating, and whilst supporting myself working in retail, I became a 'Games Maker' at the London 2012 Paralympic Games! A few days after this, I started an internship at an international HIV and AIDS charity, stunned that I had managed to bag myself this position so soon after graduating. Then just 6 months later, I applied for a job at the charity, and it is there that I am still working, feeling privileged that I have this incredible job. If I hadn't gone back to university and chosen to *carry on*, I would not be where I am now! Just as Sabrina wouldn't have made it to university too, and gained her place at Canon.

'Dance with life'

'Dance with life' – what a great motto to live your life by. Mum abided by this saying, and she even wrote it on a post-it note and stuck it on our kitchen wall. Every day we were reminded that you only get one life and it's up to you how you live it. 'Happiness is a daily decision' – another one of Mum's mottos. As she was well known for her 'dance with life' phrase, when our Uncle held a dancing competition in which there were different prizes and awards for different achievements, he gave the most entertaining award in memory of her, calling it the 'Dance with Life' award. She would have been delighted that her motto had been shared amongst others, particularly the couple who won the award.

Family life for us and Mum's side of the family has become ever closer, and all the more treasured. From seeing our grandparents little more than on special occasions, to being in touch constantly, there are some positives we've gained from the tragic loss of our Mum. The hole we all feel is filled by the new closeness of our family.

It wasn't until she passed away that we came to share her love for Max Ehrmann's 'Desiderata' poem. It hung on the wall in the study for umpteen years – not once had we read it, but had always known how much she gained from reading it. When the funeral came and we thought about how to contribute something, it was this poem that we would read aloud...

Desiderata

Go placidly amid the noise and haste, and remember what peace there may be in silence.

As far as possible, without surrender, be on good terms with all persons. Speak your truth quietly and clearly and listen to others, even the dull and the ignorant; they too have their story.

Avoid loud and aggressive persons.
They are vexations to the spirit. If you compare yourself with others, you may become vain and bitter, for always there will be greater and lesser persons than yourself.
Enjoy your achievements as well as your plans.

HELEN

Keep interested in your own career, however humble.
It is a real possession in the changing fortunes
of time. Exercise caution in your business affairs,
for the world is full of trickery.

But let this not blind you to what virtue
there is. Many persons strive for high ideals
and everywhere life is full of heroism.

Be yourself.
Especially, do not feign affection.
Neither be cynical about love, for in the face
of all aridity and disenchantment it is as
perennial as the grass.

Take kindly the counsel of the years, gracefully
surrendering the things of youth.
Nurture strength of spirit to shield you
in sudden misfortune.
But do not distress yourself with dark imaginings.
Many fears are born of fatigue and loneliness.
Beyond a wholesome discipline be
gentle with yourself.

You are a child of the universe, no less than the trees
and the stars. You have a right to be here.
And whether or not it is clear to you no doubt
the universe is unfolding as it should.

Therefore, be at peace with God, whatever
you conceive Him to be, and whatever
your labours and aspirations.

In the noisy confusion of life keep peace with your soul.
With all its sham, drudgery, and broken dreams, it is
still a beautiful world.
Be cheerful.
Strive to be happy.

Max Ehrmann, Desiderata, Copyright 1952.

For us, the words of 'Desiderata' perfectly describe Mum. They describe her character and her outlook on life, using words that go so hand in hand with her spirit. 'Peace', 'achievements', 'humble', 'strive gracefully', 'strength of spirit', 'wholesome', 'cheerful', 'strive to be happy' – this all describes Mum's positive outlook on life and her strength and determination to live life to the full. Although we never read the poem aloud on the day of the funeral, we have no regrets. We felt overwhelmed and in awe of the beauty of the ceremony. We stole the chance to keep the love for 'Desiderata' between the three of us, and now you.

Two and a half years after Mum passed away, we're still learning that 'regret' can easily creep into your mind, making you dwell on the extra time you could have spent with your loved one. It takes strength to push it out. The strength you gain from pushing it out is what ensures the memory of a loved one is a cherished one.

When we agreed to contribute to this book we thought it would be a really hard task and make us really upset, however, it has been the complete opposite. It's so easy to write about the good times we shared with Mum as they will stay with us forever.

Now we shall finish this chapter with Half Dome, Yosemite. It is there that we, our grandparents, uncle and cousin will be going to scatter Mum's ashes. What a beautiful way to celebrate our Mother's life – looking on top of the world from her favourite place.

> ### A little advice
>
> *We think the best piece of advice we can give is that life does go on. Losing someone close to you is one of the hardest things you'll have to go through, but don't forget that you also have a life to live. We feel that we're living proof of that. If your mind is in the right place, you can still succeed, even though you may be mourning. Giving everything time is important, but it's impossible to know what 'the right amount of time' is. It's different for everyone. If we hadn't pushed ourselves to revise and write dissertations so soon, even though we really didn't want to, we wouldn't be where we are today. Being content is what leads to the closest, warmest memories of your time with that person. Do not give up, do something every day that you feel would make the person you've lost proud of you. Remember the happy times that you have experienced together and suddenly the relationship you had with them seems stronger than ever.*
>
> *Carry on and dance with life… **your** life goes on.*

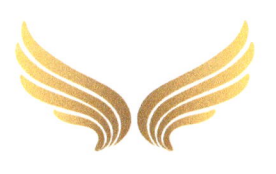

"I have been training for this all my life"

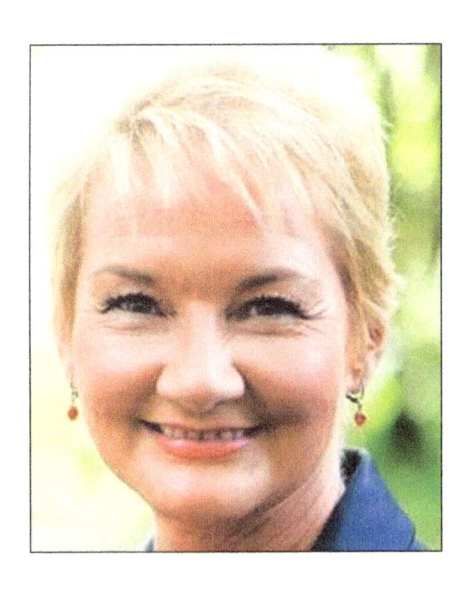

NINA JOY

Excitedly chatting to my good friend Robin Daly of 'Yes To Life' Charity in London one afternoon regarding 'Flying Free', he mentions Nina's spirited story and it resonates with me. I thought I must get in touch with this lady. Nina and I had an informal chat on the telephone: her almost sweet Yorkshire accent disarming me, whilst her unique mix of down-to-earthness, composure, ability to listen to her gut instinct in face of her serious cancer diagnosis, leading her to take decisive action, bowled me over.

Here, Nina tells her instinctive story:

I don't know how to be a patient

My professional background has been in financial services so, for the bulk of my career, that's where I have worked. I had got to quite a senior level, having a lot of responsibility and used to looking at new information. I had experience in assessing business cases, challenging what was presented or seeing if I could get corroboration for what I was being told. I am mentioning this as those are the skills I know, the skills I used when diagnosed with cancer. I don't really know how to be a patient as I have never been ill nor been in hospital. I am not a patient person and I am not very good at being told what to do. So I found what I did for a living very helpful because it gave me a framework to follow when I did not know what to do. I researched what was out there and assessed what I thought was good, what was rubbish and what was suitable for me. I was also used to taking decisions, quite big ones. I think that is something at which not everybody has practice and can find it hard. So for me, to make my decision to turn down chemotherapy, again I had some skills and practice in how I would make that decision.

"Oh do you know what? I could do that too!"

One of the biggest things that I feel many are not in touch with and need to be, is what I would call 'gut instinct'. I think people are nervous about acting on gut instinct as if it's not relevant. I think gut instinct comes from thousands and thousands of years of evolution and your own life experiences. If you are brave enough to tune into your gut instinct and follow it, I believe it takes you on the right path. I genuinely didn't know about being a cancer patient, so falling back on what I knew helped me enormously. There is no way I could have said: "Yes doctor, no doctor, three bags full doctor"; it's absolutely not in my DNA. I think that's why we should speak out, because many people have a good gut instinct and know when something they are told is the wrong thing but they either don't have the courage, the wherewithal or the confidence to actually go with it. Maybe reading our stories will give them that confidence: "Oh, do you know what? I could do that too!"

I think it's no coincidence that people who are told they have six months to live, die within six months. I have no medical knowledge at all. I literally didn't have anything to argue with, so I had to take the information the doctors gave me and, instead of taking it on board, I put it on the shelf and looked at it and thought: "So that's what they think. Right, I had better go and find out more". Professionally, there are always options, so when the doctors say: "That's the deal and there are no options", I didn't believe that to be true, however I didn't know what my options were, so had to go and seek them out. I didn't believe there were no options. When you do a business case in a commercial environment, you always put options forward. If you are going for funding for a big initiative, one of the options will always be what would happen if you did nothing.

It's only if you know what will happen if you do nothing, will you even begin to think if it's worth doing something. Well, I thought, I have one option: to do nothing. I did not believe there were no choices, but I didn't have a clue what they were, so I had to go out and look. My gut instinct kicked in for me again. I had attended a training course probably five or six years earlier, called: 'Mind Store for Business' run by Jack Black, a really amazing guy. The course was all about setting some big goals and how you could harness the power of the mind to achieve those goals. It made a huge difference to me. I did set some big goals and achieved them. While I was there Jack Black was licensing someone in Germany to use his techniques. He said this person was going to use these techniques with people who had cancer at a place called the 3E Centre! I didn't get excited at the time but thought: that's interesting. So when I was diagnosed and thought I needed to generate some options, this seemed an obvious place to start, as I knew about it already. One thing I always say to cancer patients newly diagnosed with cancer: "Hit the 'Pause' button". There seems to be an immense urgency to do something 'now' when you really haven't had the chance to know what you want to do. Even in my case, when my diagnosis was absolutely awful, you still can't tell me that taking forty eight hours to think about it will kill me or significantly affect the outcome, because it won't. I allowed myself some space to think.

An opportunity to go away for five whole weeks to concentrate on me

That's what allowed this particular memory to return: the 3E centre near Stuttgart in Germany. I googled it and found it. I looked at their website. They were still there and everything about the wording, even translated from German, absolutely spoke to me; it resonated. It was all about treating the whole person. It just sounded like that's where I needed to be. If it was up to me,

NINA

I would have packed a bag and toddled off and thought "that's it". But of course we don't live in isolation and cancer doesn't just happen to you, it happens to everyone around you. So what I experienced when I was floating the idea…I didn't know anyone who had been and had been treated there. I didn't have any guarantees, so everybody who loved me was very concerned and scared because I was gambling with my life. I probably was, to be fair. I had no precedent; all I had was my gut instinct, and I was comfortable with it. I remember telling my sister that this is what I was thinking of doing and watching the reaction on her face: "But Nina what if it's not the right decision?" It was real concern and real anguish. She wanted to support me in whatever I wanted to do but it's hard on people around you and I think we need to recognize that. Even though the norm is so bloody awful, people know people who have come through it. I think we get too attached to what the outcome is going to be. I don't know what the outcome will be if I stay here or what the outcome will be if I go there, but what I do know is, that it feels like the right course of action and that is as good as it gets. I am single with no children and I didn't have to check with a lot of people before I went. That gives you a certain freedom. I think it's very hard for those who love you. Many of my friends said you have always done things a bit differently and why would this be any different.

I decided to go to Germany for five weeks. It's a big decision. First of all, financially: you have to fund these things and that is a barrier to doing things outside the NHS from a practical point of view and going to a country where you don't understand the language. It's a big thing to do at a time when you are feeling quite vulnerable and, for me, not feeling too good physically. It's a matter of survival, when instinct kicks in: I am going to make this happen, come hell or high water. I felt excited. I felt I was getting an opportunity to go away for five whole weeks to concentrate on me. I felt really privileged. Diagnosed in August 2012, found out it had spread everywhere in September 2012 and in October I had gone. I was doing what I knew how to do.

I am not good at asking for help

Then I came back, having to incorporate it into my own life. That's when I found it really hard. Physically, I felt weak. I did a big liver cleanse when I was out there and it left me very fragile. I came home and I live on my own, so don't even have someone to bring me a cup of tea in the morning. I had to go and find where to buy the organic produce, supplies and various pieces of equipment I needed. I didn't have the energy to do that, and it really was very hard. That's another reason why, doing things the alternative way, is hard. For example, when I was first diagnosed, lots of friends offered to come and do my ironing and cleaning, thinking I was going to have chemotherapy, but because you don't lose your hair and look like you have come out of Belsen, everyone thinks you are ok. I really did not get the help that I could have done with. When I look back at my blog when I was in Germany, I can see my little pleas for help in there, but I am not good at asking for help. I am used to being independent, so found it quite hard. I can see how desperate I was for someone to come and help and take charge. But I pulled round. I muddled through really, so between November and February 2013, I carried on doing the regime and looking after myself, but, nevertheless, I was getting in a bad way.

The cancer was advancing, so I was quite poorly by March 2013 – my birthday. I really didn't think I would see another birthday, and I am not being dramatic. I did feel really ill. The tumour in my breast had really grown so near the surface and was starting to ulcerate, and a lump under my arm in my lymph system was affecting the use of my right arm. I had fluid in my lungs, so I couldn't breathe, couldn't lie down to sleep, couldn't walk very far as I was out of breath. I generally felt as though I was fading. I thought I would do what I did before. In some ways I felt *"I have been training for this all my life"*, not that I expected to get cancer, but all the experiences and skills I had learned are helping me cope with the situation I am now in. I have been here before, so I can do it again. So let's: hit that pause button....... where am I at? Let's see what there is out there.

My Cancer IFA

Again the universe came to my rescue. Something appeared under my nose which I needed. A friend of mine had been to a Professional Speaking Association meeting (of which I was a member), and updated everyone on what was happening with me. A lady whom I had never met said that she had some information that might be of use, and she sent it to my friend to pass on to me. The information she sent included a leaflet of an organization: 'Yes to Life'. So when I was thinking "what can I do now", I just rifled through all the things I had got and I found the papers that she sent to me.

I think I was looking for a Cancer IFA (who in financial services can scan the whole of the market to advise on what is best for you) as opposed to a tied agent (who can only advise on the policies of the organization they work for and are trained by. I saw doctors as tied agents). I read about Patricia Peat at Cancer Options. I remember thinking to myself: "This is it, this is my IFA"! I telephoned her and arranged to go and see her very quickly. She is based in Nottingham, which is about an hour and a half from here. I wanted to see her face to face. I was so ill. I set off to arrive there and had to have a nap on the way. I talked to her about what I had done already and what I was concerned about, and how I was now feeling physically (not good), and mentally (strong).

Your body CAN recover from where it's at

I remember she asked: "Are you totally against chemotherapy?" and I said; "Well, I am against something that wipes out my immune system, and if I have no chance of getting cured from it: it doesn't seem to make sense". And that's when she talked to me about the work of professor Vogl in Frankfurt and how he gave chemotherapy in a different manner: TACE – Trans Arterial Chemoembolization. Basically, what happens in practice is that the chemo is administered into the big artery in your groin and sent through the blood supply direct to the tumours. The idea was that I could have that for the tumour in my breast that was becoming a problem, the one under my arm and also on my lungs, as I had fluid there. She explained how much that would cost and how to travel to Frankfurt. This was exactly what I needed, as, without it, I wouldn't have lasted very long. She got me in to see him really quickly: before the end of

NINA

March 2013 I had my first treatment. I remember my sister came with me and I was very delicate and couldn't walk far. I was scared that he would take one look at the scans, and say: "I'm sorry. I'm not prepared to treat you; it's too far advanced". But he didn't, and I was incredibly relieved.

I came home from that and I slept for about a week. I think that a lot of that was the relief of knowing what I was going to be doing and that we had a plan. I carried on doing all the other stuff as well. I went back every five weeks between March and November 2013 and after every single treatment I just got better and better. By May I was pretty well: the fluid on my lungs cleared up of its own accord, the tumour in my breast shrank, the tumour under my right armpit was no longer detectable, and I could move my right arm easily. It's quite amazing really. I had the last treatment in November 2013 and, since then I have carried on doing all the other things that I need to do to look after my state of mind, toxicity, nutrition – although I am flexible about it, after all, life is for living. I have also been on Tamoxifen since November as well and various supplements. My current state of health is that, during my last visit to the hospital three weeks ago, I asked the doctor if I was in remission and he said; "Well, that would be a reasonable description of where we are at". "Good, then we will take that then" I quickly replied. From earlier scans we knew I had some cancer in my spine and in my pelvis. The latest bone scan showed that that wasn't there anymore. That's gone and, bearing in mind it's two years since I was diagnosed with cancer, I am absolutely symptom-free. I have never had a problem blood test; they have always been normal.

It's just astounding, and I think one thing that's important to get across to people with cancer, is that your body can recover from where it's at. I think it's a downward spiral that, once you get to where you are going, it can only get worse. When I was going to the hospital quite often, I used to find it a real damper on my spirits: they all seem to want to tell you what's going to happen next and all of it is awful. None of that has happened actually e.g: "We will have to drain the fluid off your lungs". Well, I have never had that done because it has cleared up. A friend of mine who is a GP asked me if I ever went to have that fluid drained. I said "no, it has cleared up". She said: "That doesn't happen", smiling at me. No, but it did.

It has given me a whole new life really!
You know they say: "Don't sweat on the small stuff". Well, I don't even sweat on the big stuff. I used to get stressed, but now, smiling serenely to myself, I think: "You know what? That doesn't really matter". You are told you have this life-limiting illness, but that gives you some freedom. This year I have been on holiday more than I have ever been in my life because I want to, and I will. Before, if I hadn't been ill, I would have thought: "I can't do that right now", for whatever reason. I don't think I have totally changed, but it has given me a whole new life really. I think it has galvanized me into action. I always used to say that one day I would write a book. Hang on, I had better make that 'one day' now! So I wrote 'The Adventures of a Cancer Maverick'. It gives you real freedom.

A little advice

1. *Hit the 'Pause' button ……………and take a little time out to digest the information and to figure out how you feel about things: not whatever everybody else is telling you to feel about things, but what you feel.*

2. *Take the time and trouble to listen to your own gut instinct, and have the confidence and courage to act on it. You are the expert on you.*

3. *Build your belief. Read stories of survivors like yours and mine. Build your belief in what you can do and what your body can do.*

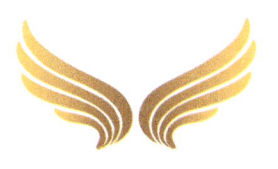

"There is ALWAYS something to be thankful for"

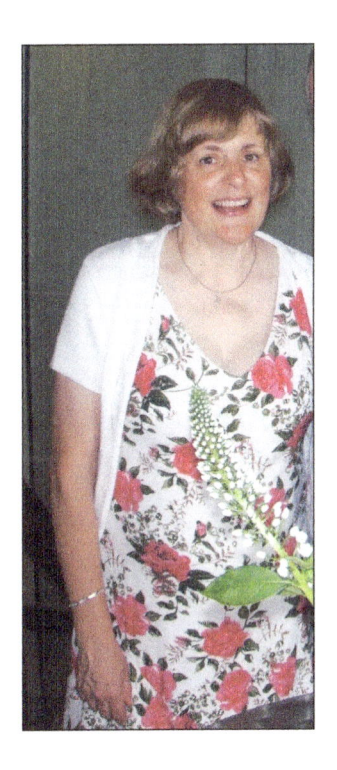

PAULINE CLARK

I first met Pauline and her partner Walter with some other friends who had just come back from The Issels Clinic in Mexico. We met in my local pub in Waddesdon, where my son and I live. It was a great and rare chance to catch up together and share our healing experiences, considering we had all gone to Mexico at different times! Pauline's attitude, in view of what she had been through, astounded me and her partner Walter's knowledge, compassion and commitment to her holistic treatment and healing was beautiful.

Here Pauline shares her remarkable story:

2008 was the year in which my life changed dramatically. I kicked off the year feeling fitter than I had done for years. I had enjoyed x-country skiing in Winnipeg over the Christmas holidays and, back at home, I'd been playing badminton and going to keep-fit classes regularly.

By the end of January, I felt a few aches in my leg, and put it down to trying too hard in a keep fit class. It carried on through February and, during a brief but enjoyable trip to Lisbon, I found some of the walking rather taxing. At Easter, my partner, Walter, and I were off on our travels again, this time to the gorgeous city of Florence for a week. As usual we walked and walked, taking in much of the fantastic artwork. We also took a train to Pisa, where we met up with an old friend and her family, who now live in Carrara, and a train to Siena where we wandered around the streets. But, as the week went on, I found myself wanting to do less walking and take longer breaks, drinking coffee and sipping Chianti, although the sights were great. On the last day, we took a train to Assisi, a place I had always wanted to visit, but I was nearly crawling by the end of the day.

Oh dear!

Once home, I went to the doctor, who diagnosed sciatica and prescribed painkillers. During the next six weeks or so, I experienced the worst and most prolonged physical pain of my life. Finally, after countless sleepless nights, I returned to the doctor, who sent me for an MRI scan. Two days after the scan I was called into the doctor's surgery and given the news that I had a tumour resting on my spinal cord. Exactly one week later, I was having a 5-hour operation; they could not remove the tumour but were taking the pressure off the spinal cord so that I wouldn't be paralysed. The surgery was successful, but involved putting two 6" titanium rods in my back to strengthen my spine.

Thankfully, I was soon walking – well, hobbling anyway – and home within 4 days, but that's not the end of the story. I was diagnosed with Leiomyosarcoma, a rare and aggressive form of cancer and I had a number of tumours in my back, pelvis and lungs. (Yes, I was shocked, and still don't know why it happened to me, given that I don't smoke, don't drink heavily, I eat healthier than most etc. But there you are. I can't complain, as I have enjoyed excellent health for most of my life.)

I was sent to a sarcoma specialist in London, who sent me for low-dose radiation in my spine, to hold off future paralysis, and spoke about possibly doing some chemo later. But she made it clear, as had other 'experts', that any treatment would only be palliative and I could not be cured. Oh dear!!

But Walter is not only an alternative health practitioner with decades of experience, but he is also a great researcher and is probably the most determined person I know. So, after days and days of on-line research he found a hospital in Tijuana, Mexico which offered alternative approaches to cancer, with a good success record. Even better, the Issels' treatment, which was offered at the hospital, has a particularly good track record with sarcoma. Initially, I was quite reticent, as I'm a pretty conventional type of person and Mexico felt like another planet to me. But the last meeting with the specialist in London made my mind up. I will always be grateful to that oncologist for her honesty in saying that the chemo wouldn't save me, because it freed me to make the decision to go to Mexico. She certainly didn't encourage my choice – I presume she saw it as a waste of money – but for me there was no point saving my money for my old age if I wasn't going to have one, so I was willing to take the chance. So off we went to the Issels Immunothapy Treatment Centre based at the Oasis Hospital in Tijuana, Mexico.

The treatment included a diet of organic fruit, nuts, beans and vegetables, with occasional organic chicken or fish – no caffeine, alcohol, refined sugar or flour; loads of supplements to support the immune system, several infusions each day of things like high-dose vitamin C, B17, "ozone", B12 injections and photopheresis treatments and several vaccines including, crucially, Coley's fluid, which stimulates the immune system. The general idea was to strengthen the whole body, especially the immune system, so that it can fight the disease itself. But the Oasis hospital, which housed the Issels clinic, offered something much broader than these physical treatments – its approach was very holistic, to strengthen the body, mind and spirit and it provided a positive, healing atmosphere.

Something I have held onto ever since

There was a little chapel in the hospital. Obviously, attendance at any of the services was optional but, early on during my 4-week stay, I thought I'd go and check out the Morning Prayer which occurred each weekday.

It started out with one of the chaplains playing a rather jolly hymn on the guitar and then the dozen or so people in the room were invited to say something they were thankful for. On this occasion I gave thanks for my friends back at home. This was followed by a couple more hymns and then a round of hugging, not something I find that easy to do with strangers, but then I'm a reserved Englishwoman! And then everyone went down for breakfast. I was left wondering why we had not prayed FOR anyone or anything – after all, the hospital was full of very sick people who surely needed all the prayers they could get. So I was not initially 'grabbed' by Morning Prayer as it was done at Oasis. However, a few days later I gave it another try and found that the format was just the same – opening hymn, everyone asked to think of something to be thankful for, more hymns, and hugs. Eventually, I began to feel a bit more comfortable with this and realised that – guess what! – being thankful every day actually helped me to feel better. And this is something I have held onto ever since – even on days when we have pain or feel down, there is always something to be thankful for – a 'phone call from a friend, something nice for lunch, the sun coming out, a funny TV programme – *there is ALWAYS something to be thankful for.* Try it and see whether it doesn't make you feel better.

After four weeks at the Oasis hospital, I returned to the UK, had a CT scan and found that my tumours had shrunk, especially those in my lungs (on which I had had no conventional treatment.) My oncologist in the UK was rather surprised and my GP said that he would not have believed it if he had not seen it for himself.

The ongoing plan was to carry on the restricted diet and supplements at home, and to have the Coley's fluid injected every other week.

'Get me outta here!'

Initially, I thought that, if I could just 'get this thing sorted', I would be returning to my old job as a primary school teacher – although, to be honest, I had reached the stage where I was no longer enjoying the job as I once had, and was sick to death of all the ridiculous paperwork. In the previous few years I had often sent up the silent prayer 'Get me outta here' – if ever there was a warning to be careful what you wish for.....So when I was advised, in early 2009, to apply for early retirement, my resistance was short-lived and half-hearted.

The first half of 2009 was a difficult time. My pain was increasing again, so that it was uncomfortable to lie down or sit for very long, and my scan in May of that year showed that my tumours had increased, despite my regular Coley's injections. Again I was offered chemo and again I refused; Walter and I were convinced that Coley's was to be a key factor in restoring my health, even though it didn't seem to be doing the job at that point and we knew that the success of Coley's was dependent on having a strong immune system, which I really did not want to compromise by having chemo. We were in touch with the doctors at Issels by e-mail and telephone and were horrified when even they suggested chemo. But we stuck with our instincts (thank goodness!) and, to this day, I have had no chemotherapy whatsoever. Instead, we asked the Issels' doctors if we should increase the dose of Coley's and they agreed that we should; we were a bit surprised that they had not suggested this to us, but it just goes to show that a patient has to sometimes take the initiative and ask the right questions. After a few, slightly larger, doses of Coley's, my pain began to go down somewhat. At this stage, none of my Coley's injections had induced any noticeable fever, and Walter, still researching, became convinced that this is what I required. I was far too scared to have a big dose of Coley's at home, so we decided to go back to Mexico, to allow me to have one under hospital supervision. We didn't go for the full month this time, for reasons of cost, but again the financial outlay felt like it would be worth every penny, if our belief about Coley's was correct – and it was. While in Tijuana, I was injected with a full 1 ml. of Coley's, under very careful supervision, and 'achieved' a fever of 38.9 deg C. On my return to the UK, I had a CT scan which revealed that my tumours had reduced by at least 50%. This time, my oncologist was amazed!

We were now gaining confidence in our own instincts with regard to my disease. Over the past few years, we have cut out some aspects of my initial 'regime' and added others when it seemed appropriate to do so. For example, while in Tijuana in 2009, we met an Australian man who had 'cured' his own oesophageal cancer through diet and wheatgrass juice. After looking into this further, we decided that I should give up juicing carrots every day and, instead, start growing and juicing wheatgrass, which is far more nutritious and great for providing an alkaline (and thus, anti-cancer) environment for the body. I can't say I love the taste, but it's bearable and, if it's keeping me well, it's OK by me. There have been many ups and downs, and my pain levels have usually been a pretty good indicator of whether the tumours were growing or shrinking. Then, about three years, into this whole adventure, we made a new 'contact' who was to make a significant contribution to my story:

Try to hold on to the fever for as long as possible

Because people I knew were surprised that I had not only survived three years but actually looked pretty perky, they mentioned me to friends of theirs who had cancer. I ended up having e-mail and telephone conversations with many people I had never met. I was happy to pass on any information which might help them, and they shared information with me. Significantly, in the space of two weeks one name came up twice, that of Doctor Henry Mannings, who had recently started up the 'Star Throwers' charity in Norfolk. For some time, Henry had been researching the literature relating to Coley's treatments (which have been used for over a hundred years, with some measure of success). He had become convinced that Coley's offered hope to certain cancer patients who maybe had less chance of success with conventional treatments, and he was brave enough to put the theory into practice in order to help people. This was wonderful news! Somebody offering Coley's treatments, not thousands of miles away in Mexico, but just 100 miles 'up the road' and, incidentally, at no cost. Not just that, but Henry was willing to administer the Coley's intravenously, which could produce a higher fever and therefore be much more effective. So, during 2011 and again in 2013, we would travel up to 'Star Throwers' once a week or, latterly, once every two weeks, for me to have a Coley's IV in order to get a fever. To try to hold on to the fever for as long as possible, I would be put to bed with four hot-water bottles under two huge duvets and after a few hours I would emerge, looking like a drowned rat from all the sweating and feeling somewhat drained. But everyone was pleased and congratulatory if I 'achieved' a high temperature. And I believe it was these fevers which have rendered my tumours inactive, so I am especially grateful to Henry and 'Star Throwers'.

So, here I am, having survived more than six years since diagnosis – that's over five years longer than I was supposed to – still juicing wheatgrass, still trying to stick to my diet to some degree, still taking lots of supplements. I am not 'cured', inasmuch as that my scans indicate I still have cancer, though my pain levels are much reduced. But, over the past six years, I have become used to 'a new normal', as Walter calls it. I am now permanently retired and my life is much slower-paced than it was. I am able to take time to enjoy doing things that I always wanted to do, especially spending hours in the garden and the allotment. We try to grow as many vegetables as we can, though we are far from being self-sufficient. Food preparation is a big priority – making nutritious organic vegetable soups from scratch, preparing salads etc. to keep my anti-cancer diet on track. We still grow wheatgrass on the windowsills and juice some every day. Although this is time-consuming, we have the time to do it and I like growing things, so it's no hardship.

Do I miss my teaching career? No, though I occasionally miss having regular contact with children. Is there anything about my past life that I miss? Of course, for example, I used to go on a walking holiday with friends every October. We would usually walk up to twelve miles a day in the glorious UK countryside; now I struggle to walk more than 3 miles at a time. I used to play badminton once a week and I would swim a mile at a time. The good news is, that I have begun to get back to these activities, although it has taken all these years to build up my strength again. Each new milestone that I reach is a real thrill for me: each time I can say "I never thought I'd be able to do that again......." The most recent of these thrills has come this year, when I find that I can swim for an hour at a time and that I am able to swim at least 1 km. It certainly hasn't happened overnight, but it gives me hope that perhaps I will, in time, be able to do other activities I used to enjoy. My next dream is to be able to return to some cross-country skiing. Meanwhile, I find I can do more and more in the vegetable plot: digging, hoeing – the works – a far cry from a few years ago when bending down to put in a few seeds was a painful and laborious undertaking, but one that I was determined to do anyway.

Life here felt like one long party!

I know that some people who get cancer feel that they go through hell with it, but for me the experience has certainly not been all bad. These last few years I have had fantastic support from friends near and far – numerous 'phone calls and visits, sometimes from very long distances, people going way out of their way to give me lifts to where I needed to go, supportive letters and e-mails. That first August, my life here felt like one long party, with all the people who called in to visit and they certainly helped to distract me from some of the physical pain. I am blessed with friends and family who were not 'frightened off' by my disease; they didn't give me a wide berth because they didn't know what to say or do. So many people 'went the extra mile' to help me in a million different ways – it's been amazing. And I know I would not be here today without the intrepid and amazing Walter, who has been on this journey with me every step of the way. I am so thankful for all of them.

A little advice

Take an active role in your treatment. Don't be rushed into having treatments you feel unhappy about and ask as many questions as you like, especially: "How effective is this treatment for my particular cancer?" Be prepared for scepticism or even outright negativity from your doctor if you choose to follow an alternative path. (One specialist told me: "There ARE no alternatives") and take responsibility for doing what your body needs in terms of rest and nutrition.

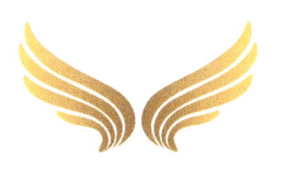

"Look up my darling, don't look back"

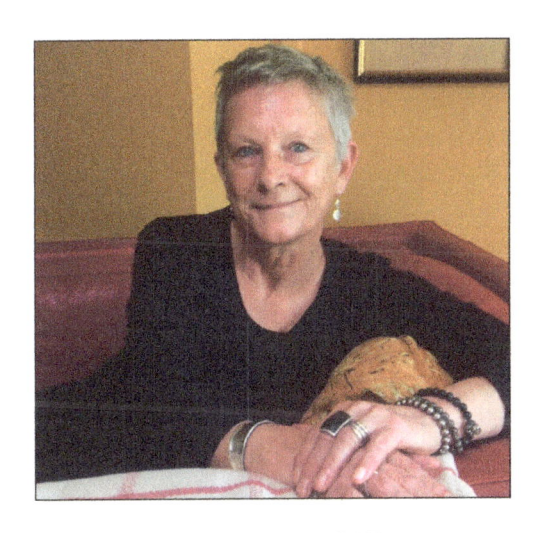

CLAIRE R. LLOYD

Claire and I met over the phone through Yes To Life Charity. We felt we knew each other already, instantly connecting with a gentle understanding and unspoken transparency. As I listened sensitively to Claire's journey, I could not understand how this lady was still standing: enduring the trauma of her own cancer, whilst bearing the pain of her daughter's cancer at the same time. Yet, a part of me did know. Having written Claire's story, I phoned one evening to check some detail which got lost in the telephone recording. Claire was sleeping and I spoke to her partner Helen. I was moved beyond words and knew I could not leave this here. The depth of Helen's commitment and love for Claire and her daughter poured out in the face of such unbelievable circumstances. The deep inner strength, compassion and love of these two amazing women abounds throughout as they bear what seems unbearable. They open their hearts to you:

The Vicar's Family!

Around the time of my birth, my father had a calling to the ministry – a draughtsman who had married my mother, who at one point saw herself as having a career in the theatre. We became 'the vicar's family' and therefore always standing as rich though not wealthy pillars of the community. Members of the community frequently visited our home at all hours and my father often disappeared into the night to help someone. The needs of others always took precedence over my own.

His first ministries were in difficult, impoverished areas and by the time I was 12, I think I had attended about 6 or 7 different schools, in a number of areas of the country. I found it difficult to invest in friendships. I was often teased and bullied at school for being a vicar's daughter. Desperately wanting to fit in, and so, as a means to impress, one day I set off the fire alarms and the school was evacuated! As a result I was sent to boarding school some miles from home. I missed my family so much and felt very isolated. On returning home at term times, my younger siblings had reformed and I no longer had a place.

Whilst we were highly regarded by the community on the outside, life was not so predictable and giving on the inside. As a charming, endearing vicar, my father was also a troubled man with periods of dark moods, retreating into himself for days on end, and self-medicating on whisky. My mother, stoic and dutiful, played the role of the vicar's wife to perfection. After all, she was on stage, but not quite in the way she had dreamed of. As a result, home always felt tense, holding a secret, almost palpable and, foreboding.

CLAIRE

Kate arrived, strong and resilient, with a thirst for life

I always wanted to have a family but the treacherous road was paved with mixed blessings. I gave birth to my first and unplanned child totally alone, booked in under a false name as my father was the Chaplain at the hospital! I married the father, more out of the fact we had a child, laying the foundations of my own family unit which meant the world to me. I became a Foster Carer, born of my empathy with those abandoned children. Two years later, little Ben was born but sadly only lived for a short time with a life-threatening disability, leaving me bereft and distraught.

I sought to fill this hole within by having another child, but I was anxious and feared I would fail to produce a child who was healthy. To my relief and complete amazement, beautiful Kate arrived, strong and resilient, with an endless thirst for life. It was difficult to believe that life could be so good to me. I was blessed. Later we adopted Joe – a troubled Afro Caribbean child – saving him from a life of domestic violence. I recall thinking: "Nobody will do that to him again". My family was complete.

Looking back for a moment, I remember meeting this young Welsh woman 'Helen', 18 years of age, the same age as me, at a party one night – a free spirit, charismatic with a touch of Celtic wildness. At this age, we were both in the process of growing up and seeking our purpose and identity. Strangely, we remained friends through our separate lives. I never really understood why, but I had a sense I could trust her. In the years that followed, we would always know when the other was in trouble, and we would see each other every 18 months or so. But I knew she was for some reason important to me and we shared many life experiences. At a young age we both understood the fragility of life.

Cwtch

After the collapse of my unsatisfying marriage when I was 31, I ventured into the unknown, with three young traumatized children.

So Cardiff became my destination and Helen once more came into my life at this scary time, pulling out all the stops and rallying all her friends to decorate my new home and help make it a home for me and the children. I learned new terms like Cwtch, that's Welsh for 'being embraced in a safe place'.

We remained friends. One night we went out dancing. and Helen turned to me and asked why we don't cwtch and teased me for my English aloofness, and so began my now 27 year relationship with my soul mate. She gave a commitment to my children and has never faltered on that and, to this day, will always help them when they need support.

I was living to work

We had both sought a career in social work, Helen in the field of child protection, and myself in the areas of children with disabilities (no surprise there) and later the fostering services. Our chosen profession was highly demanding, stressful and at times emotionally demanding. I think I was living to work and this was my vocation. Family life wasn't easy: guiding my children through the stormy waters of adolescence was at times a daily challenge.

By our late forties, both Helen and I had achieved some success in our careers: I was a director of a fostering agency and Helen an expert witness in the family courts. The children were making their own way through life. We were enjoying life and started to plan our lives without the responsibilities of children and fulfil some of the dreams we had to travel. In 2006 Helen and I became civil partners, this secured our status of next of kin and the party that followed was talked about for many weeks. Our cottage on the side of a mountain, rocked all night long until the early hours.

A journey no mother and daughter should have to make

One year later in 2007, at the age of 52, I noticed my right breast was swollen and appeared out of shape. My mother had breast cancer in her later fifties but, because she was postmenopausal, this was not viewed as a threat to my sister or me. My mother had died some years earlier but after many years of good health before succumbing to secondaries. So, without delay, I saw a specialist and, following examination, it was a cyst, sorted, moved on. The consultant advised that this may reoccur but not to worry as this might sort itself and it was quite common.

Six months later at the peak of my career, I could feel something was wrong but could not work out exactly what. In the April, I was aware of a lump in my breast and, thinking it was probably a cyst, I didn't take any notice as I had been forewarned this might happen. In August Helen urged me to go and have it checked out. I found out then that I had breast cancer in the same breast as I had the cyst. It was quite a shock. But in a strange way, as my mother had breast cancer, I wasn't totally blown out of the water. I recall Helen saying: "This will be a tough journey but we will get through it". She was my rock. When I told my daughter Kate, we urged her to get herself checked straight away. I don't know why I did that. Whilst Kate was going to her doctor, I was in hospital after having a lumpectomy. I remember lying in bed and slowly recovering when the phone rang. Kate was being sent for urgent tests, I knew we were in trouble and she was diagnosed with breast cancer. She was just 27 at the time, just six weeks after my diagnosis.

This news totally threw everything up in the air and life was becoming very dark. Knowing what I thought I knew then, it was definitely a death sentence, especially with Kate being so young at the time. Surely, this is a journey no mother and daughter should have to make. Things moved very quickly and I was haunted by the fact that when she needed me most, I was not there for her.

Nothing was certain, nothing was safe.
So Kate and I had two years of treatment. Most of this period is a blur. Emotionally, I was continually distraught to see my child having to face this and, to a greater degree, my own journey paled into insignificance

on seeing her face this. She was young, beautiful and in love. Jeff, Kate's partner of only 2 years, adapted to a very different sort of life and, seeing Kate so ill, weighed heavily on his shoulders.

I think we had about 20 operations between us, as genetic testing identified us as at high risk of recurrence. Helen cared for us both and at one time we both had double mastectomies within four days of each other. I did not have a reconstruction. My breast cancer support nurse was concerned that it might send me over the edge, as I was absolutely terrified of having something alien in me. Without barely any time to breathe, I had my ovaries out as well. Helen kept my daughter and I in touch by travelling to hospitals 40 miles apart and taking video messages between us. Nothing was certain, nothing was safe and more was to come.

"I'm out at sea on a raft and nobody can see me"
Following surgery, six months of chemo stretched ahead of us and I was terrified. I had a frightening reaction to steroids, waking up screaming the place down, overwhelmed by the thought that Kate would have to follow me having chemo. I had such a rough time that, the very thought of my precious daughter having to go through this and feel what I felt, was a nightmare. You see, with my first child dying early, Kate was my second child and I always feared losing her. When she was diagnosed, I went first and Kate would follow on 2 weeks later. Hair fallen out, dark circles around my eyes and a pale sickly pallor, following my last dose I was so weak I could no longer walk and had to be carried upstairs to bed. Kate, being younger and wearing the

cold cap every time, had managed to retain her hair and was fine on the steroids, but chemo takes you to a dark place and I remember asking her how she felt, and she replied: "like I'm out at sea on a raft and nobody can see me, and I am alone". I sunk to rock bottom, both physically and mentally, and had to build myself up again. My whole focus was on Kate, so I didn't really think about my own traumatic experience of cancer.

Look up my darling, don't look back

After two years, we started our journey of recovery. For Helen and Jeff, they had witnessed this and felt powerless to stop us hurting. It affects all those around you. Helen, little known to me at the time, used to keep her sanity by writing late at night and I later found she had written this:

Looking Back

Looking back in silence,
Nothing was easy, nothing was sacred.
Clouds of despair descended and covered our world.
Fear made us run for safety, only to
find there was none.
Life cast us aside to face a dark and violent rage
Trembling with fear, gasping for air,
we walked into the rain.

Standing alone, rising cold waters surrounded you.
You struggled to keep your head above
the tide of despair.
Slashed and poisoned, it threatened your
very existence.

CLAIRE

The light faded from your eyes,
as the battle within raged.
Pain etched across your face and
only your shadow remained.

The storms slowly subsided and
fragments of light reappeared.
Life had not forsaken you but taken
you on a journey to the edge.
Exhausted, you turned to see
that we had all made it through.
Then screams of relief bellowed from
the depths of your soul
And your tears ran freely as you began
your long journey home.
The light grew stronger and warmed
your tired limbs

And you stooped to pick up the fragments
of your broken life,
Some bent out of shape, some lost forever,
some yet to retrieve.
Struggling to rebuild the pieces, not
recognizing their new form,
And the ashes from your battles stared
back from your scars.
Growing into new skin, fumbling to
repair broken parts,
Straining to find the way back and make
sense of your new life,
Would you recognize your home when you saw it?
It's not changed but somehow different,
somehow older.
But it's still a place to heal and be healed.

Having looked back in silence, I turn to
face the road ahead:
Waiting for your return, longing to walk
by your side,
I witnessed your pain and suffering, now
I will lead you away
I lie next to you as you sleep, aching to
hold you in my arms again,
And gently whisper:
"look up my darling, don't look back".

We started our own laughter workshop at home

Like everybody else, I had the desire to get back to normal afterwards. I went back to work but I was highly anxious. Things never really eased up. We had about a month when we thought: "we are ok". Then Kate started having symptoms and further investigations. I was forever on edge. In those hard days I did manage to have jokes with others about being lucky and being thankful. When things got really bad, Helen and I started our own laughter workshop, practising laughing at home, and we did begin to laugh again and I never thought we would. Helen was my amazing rock: "It will pass and nothing stays the same". We checked out what is real, what is true and discussed our fears. We accepted that some days are down days and that it's okay to cry and let out those toxic feelings. I started going to all sorts of workshops on mindfulness which didn't seem to do any good at the time.

'I am frightened I have got cancer again'

In June 2013, five years after my first diagnosis, I sort of felt a bit sick but didn't take much notice as I was trying to get my career back in line. I had some 'not very wells' and woke up one day with a pain quite high up, very different from anything I had ever experienced. I began to go downhill and quickly took myself off to my see my GP. He didn't think there was anything much wrong and said: "You have a history of depression since being diagnosed", implying it was all in my mind when I was really ill. I felt patronized and burst into tears: "I am frightened I have got cancer again" which I hadn't thought of until that moment. That evening I said to Helen: "I really don't feel very well at all. I think I need to go and see the emergency doctor". As I walked into his surgery he said: "you are a very nasty colour" and arranged a blood test immediately. The results came back: I had shadows on my liver suggesting I had secondary liver cancer. My oncologist confirmed the diagnosis. I was too shocked to put this into words, but had good loving people around me. A few weeks later, fate dealt a very cruel blow, my beautiful daughter Kate was also diagnosed with secondaries – bone metastases. Shock and waves of sadness and despair revisited me, but this time I had tools to help me through, keep in the present, let the tears out and accept reality and not become overwhelmed with fear. This helped me to adjust to our new position in a much shorter time frame. Back to the basics I had learned: be kind to myself and allow myself to be vulnerable, which is quite different from self-pity.

Treated for free

An American friend Shirley was into alternative stuff and impacted my thinking. She did some research and took me along to see a naturopath, Keith Jones. Ensconced in his quaint old office with its battle- weary worn leather couch, he treated me for free, giving me lots of tests. I did not question too much, just going with it. I followed his warm advice along with other golden nuggets of information that I picked up en route, changing my diet radically to an alkaline-based regime. I didn't feel any worse. When I went for a check-up 3 months later everything was the same, but the next check-up revealed that my tumours had started shrinking and they have continued to do so to the extent that my oncologist is puzzled.

I started to change my life in many ways, getting rid of toxic relationships, where people can be either radiators or drains. I realise now that I do not sweat the small stuff. Thoughts are just thoughts, it doesn't mean it's all true. I have learned to flip the coin and look at the positive, not the negative. I have to listen to myself. It's a kind of acceptance of my situation. I never thought I would get to this point. I thought I would be in a psychiatric hospital by now. I am surprised that I can be happy, I can laugh. It's probably since my second diagnosis, when I fully realized, for the first time, that maybe I am not going to have to watch my daughter die, maybe I am going to die first. It dawned on me that I must watch that I didn't set myself up to be a role model: so if Kate is still going, then I have to keep going! I think I was in a bit of victim mode.

You are witnessing the deconstruction of yourself
The NHS pushes you into victim really. Looking back on what I have been through, I can see why:

At the point of being diagnosed with breast cancer, the strongest emotion that rises from within you is fear,

fear that fills your every waking moment of each day and is so powerful you will do anything to take that away. So you follow and trust, with the innocence of a child, those who offer some hope and release from the darkness that surrounds you.....the victim has been created. You are stripped to the waist and your breasts are prodded and poked by numerous faceless men and then drawn on with felt pen. You are witnessing the deconstruction of yourself, without any resistance, your only defence is to weep. Now, like a lamb to the slaughter, you are cut, poisoned and burnt....but this is the promised cure, be grateful to be alive…Why am I on the edge of despair? After the cure has been completed, when you look in the mirror, you hardly recognise yourself, no hair, dark circles around your eyes. A relaxing soak in the bath is no more; it is now a trauma, as you pick up the courage to look down at the body you once knew so well. Who am I? There is no going back.

There are lots of people bearing things much worse

Accepting that suffering is a part of life is important: if you don't suffer you don't feel the other side which is joy. Being aware of being positive, I was busy searching for the first signs of Spring. It's really hard when I do see Kate, about once a month, because I am like a scanner myself. We message each other every day. I think this has had to happen and we both knew without realizing it: we both had to get on with our own lives. If we see each other, the reality hits me, as I am usually away in my own world. Then Kate mentions that she is going for a brain scan: I just feel her pain and think I can't bear it ......but I do bear it. There are lots of people bearing things much worse. When I am down, Helen and I go for a drive to change the scene. I have a couple of inspirational books too. Maybe I have to come to terms with what happens to us when we die. I am not fearful of death itself but of the process. I also have a sense of a great reunion in the sky. I have read too many things that all point in the same direction not to believe that. So I certainly feel there is something much more. I have also turned myself inside out about things in the past. Sometimes I wonder if I could be doing penance, from past generations, not my fault. So I have examined every detail of what I have done wrong. I haven't been a person who has always done right. This journey is a bit like an endurance test: just how much can you endure really? This can blow your head off as you have to find reasons to carry on living. But I do find those reasons and feel blessed that I am so loved. I have just really started looking after myself at 60!

Learning to dance in the rain

For sure, there are dark times on this breast cancer journey, so I am going to learn how to 'dance in the rain'. The compassion and empathy I had shown others was now focused on me. I would not entertain the idea of the 'battle with cancer' or the term 'survivor' – where does that leave those who die from this disease: failures! No, I needed to enable my body to help heal itself and that meant a total overhaul of my habits, lifestyle and the connection with myself.

Throughout my life, anxiety had been my constant companion, so meditated to calm my head chatter.

CLAIRE

Learning that, however bad things seem, nothing stays the same, that I would move through it, learning to identify reality from fear and to keep things simple. Some friends can't stay around, don't judge them, for others will appear and surprise you.

Our large garden was overgrown with brambles and really in a bad state. And our two dear friends Kath and Shirley lovingly gave up their Sunday afternoon every week for months on end to devote themselves to totally transforming our 200ft nagging source of worry into a healing, peaceful oasis. We never asked them. Afterwards we would sit around eating and celebrating heart-felt friendship. We fondly refer to this as our 'gardening club'.

Listen to your body if you feel tired in the company of other people; it is because energy is being taken from you. Stay around those who make you feel energized, I term this habit as identifying people as either drains or radiators: stick with the radiators, your energy is limited.

Learning to listen to my body: what did I need? Stop and think before making a decision to accept invitations: maybe I really need to rest.

I kept a routine: get up and shower. I would not be seen as the victim, but also needed to accept afternoon naps, which became treasured space. I researched diet: cleared the house of all harmful products, learned that oestrogen, my enemy, was labelled under all types of obscure names. Sugar was also out: having been a bit of a chocoholic, it was like saying goodbye to an old friend. I started juicing and eating only organic food.

Treats came in many different forms: pedicures and facials became, and still are, things that make me feel better. I found the power of distraction very useful, stopped listening to the news and all the sad events in the world, about which I could do nothing. Instead, I read books for pleasure, usually 2 or 3 a week. That's my private pleasure, where I can venture outside my own existence.

Then, time to look at the big wide world out there, all the trips I promised I would do one day. Well, one day was here and now. We went to New York shopping on 5th Avenue, Iceland to see the Northern Lights, and then the magic of Morocco to smell the spices and see the brilliant colours.

This was the new me, old habits gone, life was for living now. When I feel sad I cry, this allows me to laugh when happy and see the joy in the world around.

Be gentle with my little girl

Sadly, two weeks after agreeing to write my story, Kate has been diagnosed with extensive brain metastases. So I sit before you, typing my story. To say I am not heartbroken is an understatement. I look around, my tool bag ready, friends, my partner, standing firmly by my side to go on a journey that every parent dreads, the loss of your child. I have to flip the coin: the other side of my present challenge is that I am well enough to be her mother, whereas, before, I was too ill. I will nurture, soothe and take care of her. I am her mother once more. Whatever spiritual beliefs I have, all I ask is: "Be gentle with my little girl, as I walk her home to meet with you".

Shadows

We are in the twilight zone now: the space
between the night and day.
The long warm days of summer and
the freshness of the spring, where the rain
and sunshine dances all over your senses,
are behind us now.

The reassuring sound of the dawn chorus
is now quiet, replaced by slowly forming shadows.
As the sun drops from the sky, the light cools to
prepare us in a kind of limbo as we grow fearful
of the long night ahead.

We want those hot summer days to last,
just a little longer,
We want the birds to sing to out loud
to welcome the day.
As the darkness of the long night ahead beckons,
we start to get used to this dimmed light and for now
we are learning to play in the ever changing light of
the shadows.

A little advice

If anxiety is your uncomfortable companion, ease your mind by meditating.

Be aware of, however bad things seem, nothing stays the same and you CAN move through it.

Keep things simple and identify reality from fear.

Don't judge some of your friends who can't stay around; others will appear and surprise you.

Stay around those who make you feel energized, not drained.

Stop and think before accepting invitations: maybe you need to rest.

Allow yourself to have your feelings, even the painful ones.

Keep a healthy routine: rise and shine, accept and treasure afternoon naps.

Clear your home of all harmful products.

Stop sugar and start juicing and eating organic food.

Treat yourself to what makes you happy: pedicures and facials make me feel better.

Listen to good news and read books for pleasure, stepping out of your own existence.

Laugh out loud and enjoy the good times.

Having a sense of purpose helps you discover parts of yourself you didn't know, saving you from becoming swamped by the all-encompassing challenges of this dis-ease.

In short, give yourself the life you truly deserve.

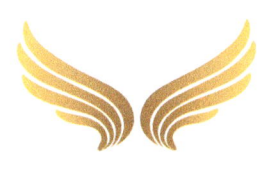

"I needed cancer in my life to heal completely"

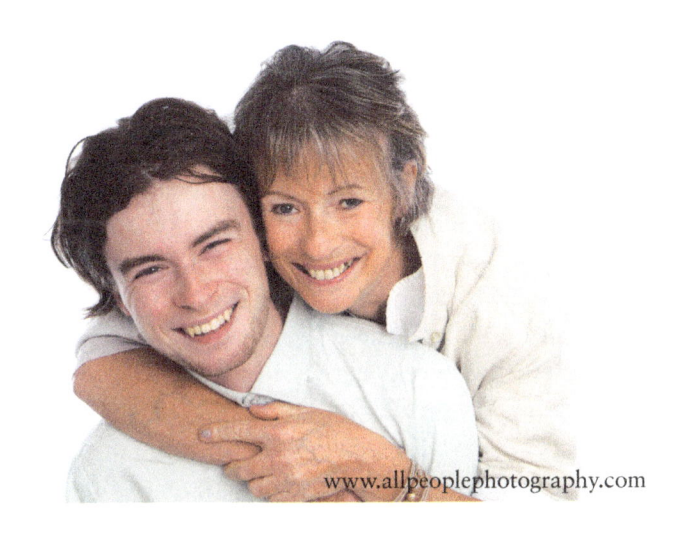

JACINTA MCSHANE – AUTHOR AND THRIVER

Originally when thinking about creating: 'Flying Free', I had not envisaged including a chapter on my journey with my son, having already written my story a few years earlier: 'Hidden Gifts – an abuse survivor's triumph through cancer'. However as these wonderful stories flowed through me, I felt differently.

Here I look back on my life-changing, enlightening, blessed journey over the past 11 years with endless hope, limitless love for my son and complete faith in the Godness within:

Jacinta

Diagnosed with breast cancer eleven years ago, I never thought I would be alive today, to be in this position: to be able to and want to look back on the blessings of cancer in my life.

It was absolute hell to start with in 2004. I thought it was the end. I fell into a million pieces which I think now was my saving grace and the beginning of an incredible journey. I was terrified of everything, absolutely everything. I felt that my back was broken, I could shoulder no more. I was falling apart, shattering from the inside out. Isn't it amazing the power within that single word 'cancer'? A few weeks earlier I felt fine. Nothing much had changed physically in those few preceding weeks, yet my whole world came crashing down, nonetheless. Unbeknown to me, here was my divine beginning to heal! Thank God, I did not try to keep everything together!

Looking back, I can see what happened: upon hearing the word 'cancer' for the first time, it meant instant death to me, taking me back to my childhood. This triggered an immediate, strong, innate response within my body to live and never be a victim again. This disease was the physical manifestation of my need to heal emotionally and spiritually from a very long time ago. Diagnosis gave me the jolt that I desperately needed. I grabbed that opportunity with everything I had to live, especially for my son.

Whilst my journey has been challenging and traumatic at times, the closer I came to confronting deep-seated emotional pain, the easier it became. I have never felt that I have been through that much physically, though my friends might disagree. I felt everything emotionally – an explosive release of past and present. I remember saying to my surgeon after my mastectomy eleven years ago: "the more of my body you remove, the more I find inside!" He did look perplexed, poor man! In the midst of raw vulnerability, those surprising words popped out with sheer delight.

I would never have believed that cancer could transform our lives so amazingly: from selling our home, moving to wonderful Waddesdon, being made redundant, travelling the whole way to Mexico for immunotherapy treatment to complement my treatment here, writing my own story in 'Hidden Gifts', speaking here and there, and now writing this book inspired by the incredibly spiritually healing stories of remarkable others who have crossed my path.

Prior to cancer, life was about 'getting'. Post cancer, life was and is all about 'giving'. Gosh! 'Giving' is so much easier and effortless than 'getting' ever was and gives me so much more!

I have always believed that it doesn't really matter what drugs or treatment I am given, if I am not 100% behind it, then it won't make much of a difference. Some part of me always knew that I needed to heal within myself. This was key to my recovery and has proven to be so. Ignoring that yearning would have been disastrous.

Why let your body be treated and expect tough drugs to do it all? That's a tall order. Those drugs do not know us, they do not know our bodies, how we feel, how we think, how we are coping. We are living, thinking, feeling 'hosts' and cancer is systemic, affecting our entire systems. It seems vital that we play our part in our complete healing. After all, doctors can treat us. We may like to think they are GODS but even THEY cannot heal us – that part is mostly down to us: our involvement, our will power, our hope, our love and our complete faith.

Thank you Geraldine (see Dedication) for your life-changing words as I approached surgery each time: "You are more than your body, Jacinta". I realise now that being at my most vulnerable, stripped bare of all my learned defences, my spirit could really hear you.

*Then your **light** will break forth like the dawn, and your **healing** will quickly appear; then your righteousness will go before you, and the glory of the Lord will be your rear guard.*

Isaiah 58:8

I have written my own raw, healing story: 'Hidden Gifts- an abuse survivor's triumph through Cancer' published in 2010 (see sample chapter towards the end). This gives you the guts and bare bones of my journey, physically, emotionally and spiritually – a rollercoaster of ups and downs, shocks and thrills, fears and hopes, darkness and incredible light which shines brighter every day.

My biggest challenges have been coping with my fears, not of death as you might imagine, but of the uncertainty of treatment, the uncertainty of the future, my extreme fear of needles, my concern for my son: mostly primal fears. Now as time goes on and I come through more challenges, I feel that I am growing bigger and bigger, taller and taller inside: fear gently giving way to growing trust in myself and others, guilt giving way to self-forgiveness, anger giving way to love. I am beginning to see love around me, in the most unexpected and unlikely places.

Yes I dip, yes I wobble and yes fear consumes me at times, but not for long these days – love becoming stronger than any fear. As my understanding oncologist often gently utters: "In the grand scheme of things, Jacinta, this is not too bad." That phrase: 'in the grand scheme of things' has followed me religiously through the years, and what a balancer it is. It certainly brings things into perspective and pulls me out of the sinking sands of disease. Oh to be out of my own way! Oh to be more than my own body! This is what 'flying' is all about!

As Marianne Williamson says beautifully in her book 'A Return to Love', "the purpose of our lives is to give birth to the best which is within us." I can fly. I would have it no other way.

A little advice

This might be our last stand, as it were, so why not give it our 'all': dive in and discover what our cancer is really telling us. What have we got to lose! The chances are that we may have lost it already, without knowing.

I believe that it can take years and years for tumours to develop, years and years of bad habits, excesses, addictions, poor nutrition, lack of self-love etc. Now we can give ourselves the chance that our spirits have been crying out for – hope, healing and nurture. We CAN create our own miracle

By diving in, I found pure light. Each day becomes lighter and lighter and I am truly grateful for every moment. I am blessed.

Join me!

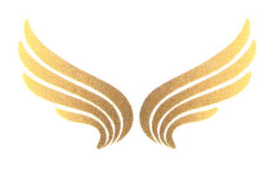

*'Cancer can be the 'beginning' of us,
NOT the 'end' of us'*

The Beginning

Cancer has a wonderful way of stripping us bare of all our various roles in life, whether we are parents, grandparents, sons or daughters; whether we are employed, self-employed, unemployed or retired; whether we are married, widowed, divorced or single. Cancer strips us bare of our possessions, whether we own our own home, have a mortgage, rent, live in a large house, a small house, an apartment in an affluent area or a poor area, and the list goes on. Cancer changes our thinking, changes our attitudes, and changes our priorities. Cancer is about our 'insides' not our 'outsides'. It brings us to ourselves, whoever we are, wherever we are. If we look in and listen, we come out beautiful and glorious.

In prayers one morning in this hospital in Mexico, I remember meeting this tall, handsome, eloquent, articulate man who was very charming. He told me that he was all right from the neck down! He proudly, if not somewhat arrogantly, told me that he was a director of his own high profile consultancy in New York, married with children, wealthy with a large social circle of influential connections, huge estate, fleet of cars etc.

Later, having lunch together, I asked him about his cancer. He was diagnosed with throat cancer a month ago and given a few months to live! Just prior to coming into hospital, he had stepped down as Company Director and told his friends. Slowly, over lunch, his ego slipped away, unmasking his fear, insecurity and fragility. Whilst this was heart-rending, it was also beautiful. He began facing himself. None of his former achievements or accomplishments mattered now. This was his blessed 'beginning'.

It's amazing how our spirits can soar in the face of crisis. This is a powerful personal choice showing the potential of man that lies deep within everyone of us. These 'thrivers' have given themselves 'life' and we can all do this for ourselves. We have the power within us to heal ourselves from the inside out, allowing ourselves to be all we can be. We gain a clarity that enables us to see beyond, we live life in a whole new fulfilling way. Just imagine how different our world would be if we all allowed our spirits to soar in the course of everyday living!

I have found writing, listening and gathering these wonderful stories together, unexpectedly lightening and fulfilling; lifting me up, all binds dropping away and light shining everywhere.

We are never our 'ends', we are always our 'beginnings'.

We can fly!!!!

Dear Jesus, help us fly,
fly from the deepest part of ourselves.
Help us bathe in
Your glory,
Your magnificence,
Your splendour.
Build us up to be almighty,
In Your image,
Powerful in your presence,
Teeming with love and hope and the strength
to heal the whole world.

Onward!

As you have read the inspiring words of each person's journey with cancer, I pray that you will have been inspired, not only by the courage and determination of each one of them in their own particular battle, but also by the power of spiritual healing: the indescribable power and love of God!

Elaine Ferguson, Editor

All The little advice

Michelle

"I could find joy in the simplest of things and I never stopped being in awe of the beauty and majestic power of nature in all its glory".

Advice:

Nothing in life can prepare you for dealing with this, so be patient and do what is right for you and your partner. Although it is tempting to talk about the past and happy occasions, I found that this made Dan uncomfortable and a little sad, as did talking too much about the future. Stay in the present moment and enjoy every minute of your time together. Now is the time for 100% unconditional love. Don't be afraid.

Jay

"I thanked God for this pain"

Advice

I had my last session of chemo that month – less than 6 months later I was told I was clear and I've been clear ever since. I never once owned it. I never once referred to being ill as 'my' cancer. I told the doctors, referring to it as such, too. It may have been there, but it wasn't there to stay.

Iain

"If cancer is a messenger, it has an urgent message; if I can interpret that, I stand some chance of putting it right."

Advice

So keep positive, think of the best, believe in yourself, and stay well! 'Finally, brethren, whatsoever things are true, whatsoever things are honest, whatsoever things are just, whatsoever things are pure, whatsoever things are lovely, whatsoever things are of good report; if there be any virtue, and if there be any praise, think on these things'.

Philippians 4:8

Glenn

"I had to go forward from here"

Advice

Our aim in sharing our experiences with you was:

Firstly, to underline that our bodies are capable of beating even the diseases our medics deem to be incurable, without THEIR intervention.

Secondly, to let you know what we did, so that you have some immediate practical course of action to start on while you do your own research. Each of us has to take responsibility for our own health and well-being, rather than leaving it in the hands and minds of others.

Consequently, we suggest that you seek out books and websites yourself, by simply asking around or typing in your particular health concern into your web browser. You will be amazed at the enormous quantity of information that is freely available, and how often 'just the right book' falls into your lap. We encourage you to read and research for yourself until, like us, you become convinced that you or your loved one can improve your health by aiding your body to function at its best.

We hope that somewhere amongst our stories, you will find the inspiration and/or information you need to create your own 'wellness miracle'.

Marilyn

"This is not a death sentence, just something that needs to be worked through, and my body's way of letting me know I need to make some SERIOUS changes."

Advice

If I were asked to sum up our approach it would be: "Re-evaluate and question everything – your understanding of life, any treatment advice given to you, your diet, lifestyle, family, work, recreation time – looking specifically for stressing/unhelpful factors, and change/improve things wherever possible, because the very act of taking control, even over little things, empowers you energetically, to say nothing of changing your body chemistry in ways that allow your body to heal – and last but not least, look for the gift in EVERYTHING!"

Gordon

"I am now flying and free of the chains that had been holding me down. Life is exciting"

Advice

1. *When diagnosed, don't panic. Most people have time to put a plan together. You are now number one on your priority list: it's all about what <u>you</u> want from now on in.*
2. *Get hold of at least one person who is knowledgeable and trustworthy to act as a cancer life coach with whom you can to talk through everything and anything. Most importantly, try to work out why you have cancer. This will help you immensely on your journey.*
3. *Don't commit to any treatment just because someone said you should do it. Do it because it either makes sense to you or it actually makes you feel better emotionally or physically (or both).*
4. *Don't submit to any person. I recommend you have your faith only in Jesus Christ. Find a Christian Church that relates to you and declares that it's God's will to heal you.*
5. *Don't stress about getting everything right at the beginning. It's a journey where you come across people and treatments along the road. Some you*

take on board, others you have to discard for the journey. Value those people who come to you and stay with you for the duration of your journey.
6. *Celebrate every little success. Discard any news or person who says you can't do anything about the cancer. It's a massive lie. Seek to live only in truth.*

Helen

"I always knew there was so much more!"

Advice

We think the best piece of advice we can give is that life does go on. Losing someone close to you is one of the hardest things you'll have to go through, but don't forget that you also have a life to live. We feel that we're living proof of that, if your mind is in the right place, you can still succeed, even though you may be mourning. Giving everything time is important, but it's impossible to know what 'the right amount of time' is. It's different for everyone. If we hadn't pushed ourselves to revise and write dissertations so soon, even though we really didn't want to, we wouldn't be where we are today. Being content is what leads to the closest, warmest memories of your time with that person. Do not give up, do something every day that you feel would make the person you've lost proud of you. Remember the happy times that you have experienced together and, suddenly, the relationship you had with them seems stronger than ever.

*Carry on and dance with life... **your** life goes on.*

Nina

"I have been training for this all my life"

Advice

1. *Hit the 'Pause' button ....and take a little time out to digest the information and to figure out how you feel about things: not whatever everybody else is telling you to feel about things, but what <u>you</u> feel.*
2. *Take the time and trouble to listen to your own gut instinct, and have the confidence and courage to act on it. You are the expert on you.*
3. *Build your belief. Read stories of survivors like yours and mine. Build your belief in what you can do and what your body can do.*

Pauline

"There is ALWAYS something to be thankful for"

Advice

Take an active role in your treatment. Don't be rushed into having treatments you feel unhappy about and ask as many questions as you like, especially: "How effective is this treatment for my particular cancer?" Be prepared for scepticism or even outright negativity from your doctor, if you choose to follow an alternative path. (One specialist told me: "There ARE no alternatives").

And take responsibility for doing what your body needs in terms of rest and nutrition.

ALL THE LITTLE ADVICE

Claire

"Look up my darling, don't look back"

Advice

If anxiety is your uncomfortable companion, ease your mind by meditating.

Be aware of, however bad things seem, nothing stays the same and you CAN move through it.

Keep things simple and identify reality from fear.

Don't judge some of your friends who can't stay around; others will appear and surprise you.

Stay around those who make you feel energized, not drained.

Stop and think before accepting invitations: maybe you need to rest.

Allow yourself to have your feelings, even the painful ones.

Keep a healthy routine: rise and shine, accept and treasure afternoon naps.

Clear your home of all harmful products.

Stop sugar and start juicing and eating organic food.

Treat yourself to what makes you happy: pedicures and facials make me feel better.

Listen to good news and read books for pleasure, stepping out of your own existence.

Laugh out loud and enjoy the good times.

Having a sense of purpose helps you discover parts of yourself you didn't know, saving you from becoming swamped by the all-encompassing challenges of this dis-ease.

In short, give yourself the life you truly deserve.

Jacinta

'I needed cancer in my life to heal completely'

This might be our last stand, as it were, so why not give it our 'all': dive in and discover what our cancer is really telling us. What have we got to lose! The chances are that we may have lost it already, without knowing.

I believe that it can take years and years for tumours to develop, years and years of bad habits, excesses, addictions, poor nutrition, lack of self-love etc. Now we can give ourselves the chance that our spirits have been crying out for – hope, healing and nurture. We CAN create our own miracle

By diving in, I found pure light. Each day becomes lighter and lighter and I am truly grateful for every moment. I am blessed. Join me!

References

Issels Integrative Immuno-Oncology: www.issels.com
The Oasis of Hope Hospital: www.oasisofhope.com
SPACE: www.aylesburychurches.org/st-mary-the-virgin/space
Aylesbury Town Chaplaincy: www.aylesburytownchaplaincy.co.uk
The Pink Ladies' Breast Cancer Support Group: www.pinkladies.org.gg

Chapter 2 Michelle

www.clipperroundtheworld.com

Chapter 3 Jay

www.globalretreatcentre.org
'A Return to Love' by Marianne Williamson

Chapter 4 Iain

Iain's Blog www.iaincarstairs.wordpress.com
Dr. Bruce Lipton www.brucelipton.com
The Budwig Diet www.budwigdiet.co.uk

Chapter 5 Gordon

Robin Daly: www.yestolife.org.uk
Professor Thomas Vogl: www.radiologie-uni-frankfurt.de
Riviera Life Church, Torquay, Devon: www.rivieralife.co.uk
    www.en.leading-medicineguide.com/Specialist-Radiology-Frankfurt-Prof-Vogl
Dr Stephen Hopwood at the Arcturus Cancer Care Clinic in Totnes
    www.arcturusclinic.co.uk

Chapter 7 Marilyn

The Oasis of Hope Hospital: www.oasisofhope.com
'Biology of Belief' by Bruce Lipton

Chapter 8 Helen

Bosom Friends Cancer Support Group www.bosomfriends.org.uk
Breast Friends' Cancer Support Group www.breastfriends-aylesbury.org.uk
Cancer Research Relay for Life: www.relayforlifeaylesbury.org
Florence Nightingale Hospice: www.fnhospice.org.uk
'Desiderata' by Max Ehrmann

Chapter 9 Nina

Patricia Peat www.canceroptions.co.uk
Robin Daly: www.yestolife.org.uk
Professor Vogl:
    www.en.leading-medicine-guide.com/Specialist-Radiology-Frankfurt
3e centre: www.3e-centre.com/
'The Adventures of a Cancer Maverick' by Nina Joy available on
    www.amazon.co.uk
'How to be a Cancer Maverick' by Nina Joy coming out soon

Chapter 10 Pauline

Issels Immuno-Oncology Centre www.issels.com
Dr. Henry Mannings: www.starthrowers.org.uk

Chapter 11 Claire

Keith Jones Naturapath – Four Winds Healing Centre Tel: 01446 420155

Suggested Reading

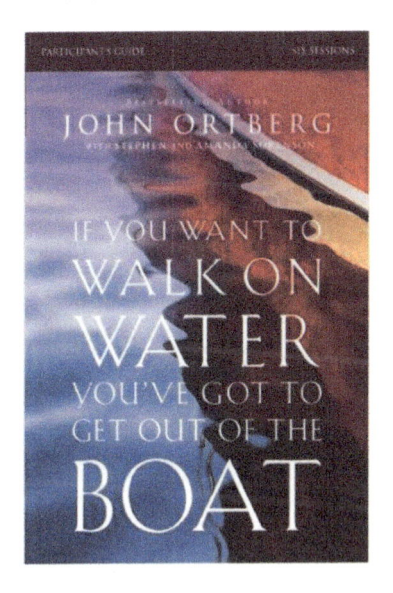

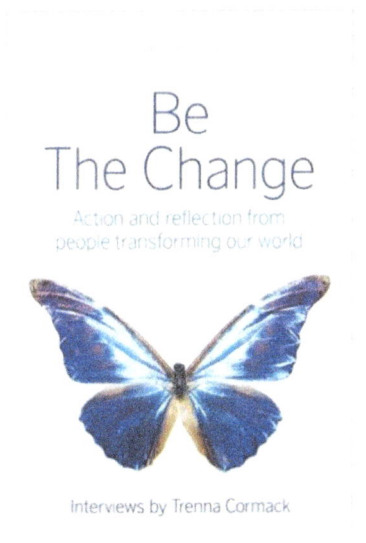

JOHN ORTBERG

IF YOU WANT TO WALK ON WATER YOU'VE GOT TO GET OUT OF THE BOAT

Be The Change

Action and reflection from people transforming our world

Interviews by Trenna Cormack

(Further suggested reading in 'References')

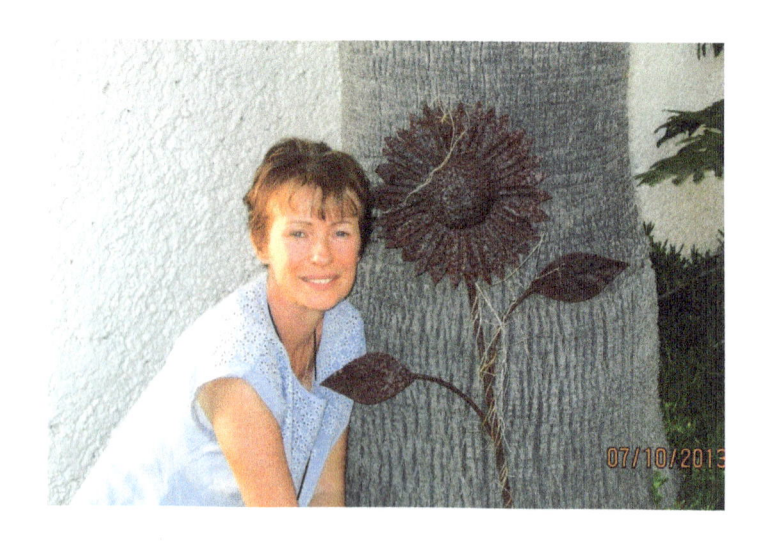

Celebrate Your Journey

If you would like to have your own book about your journey (or your loved one's) through cancer but don't feel you are able to put it into written words, I would love to help bring your personal story into print for you.

I can come to you and listen to your story, recording it and later transcribing it into print, complete with special photographs and/or illustrations that you may like to include. We can work together to bring your story to light in the way that you would like and mark your triumph through cancer. You can email me on: hiddengifts@hotmail.co.uk

God bless

Jacinta

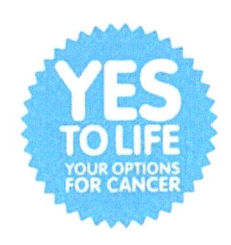

Help 'Yes to Life' to help others like they help me

'Yes to Life' is a charity that supports people with cancer in the UK in taking an integrative approach to their treatment.

Integrative Medicine is a broad approach that combines the best of Complementary & Alternative Medicine with standard treatments, to widen choice, extend care and improve results.

'Yes to Life' offers support to people with cancer who want to take a proactive role in their treatment. We help open up choices and support people in finding a way forward that is right for them.

"I remember first meeting Robin Daly – Chairman of 'Yes to Life' Charity, in London. I was moved and strengthened by his own story of his daughter Bryony, and instantly knew then that here was someone who had stepped forward and would help me in the way I needed. 'Yes to Life' has supported me solidly and consistently in ways no other charity would. Their broad knowledge of Integrative Medicine, precise information when I needed it, and practical financial support, has helped me source the complementary treatment I need to be truly well."

http://yestolife.org.uk/supportus/donate.html

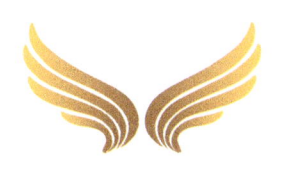

Hidden Gifts

A Preview

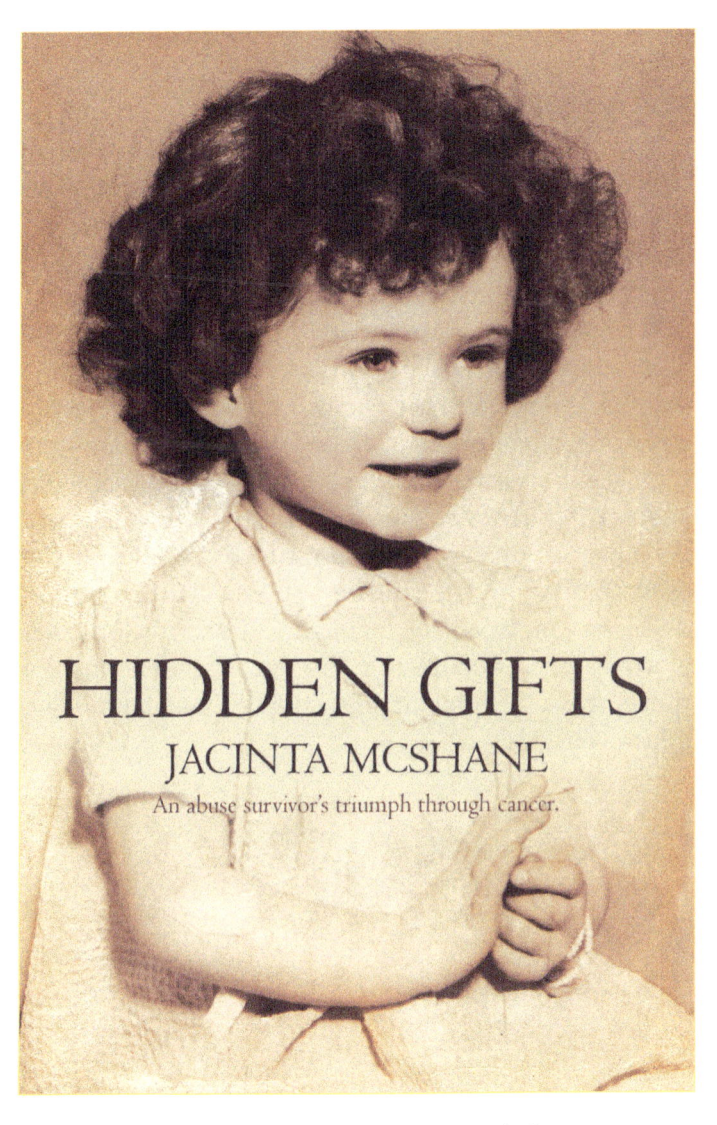

HIDDEN GIFTS
JACINTA MCSHANE
An abuse survivor's triumph through cancer.

*'I needed Cancer in my life to
heal completely'*

This book is dedicated to all those children who once
were, who need to find their voices to heal

Staring death in the face of a cancer diagnosis throws the world of this professional single mother and her nine year old son into sheer chaos. As her world begins to fall apart, she sinks uncontrollably into the suppressed, agonising pain of her traumatic childhood at the hands of her abusive parents. With a relentless determination not only to survive but to live life fully in every way, she painstakingly claws her way back from her past finding the courage to confront her worst fears. This is a true story of past and present, emotional, physical and spiritual healing written with raw emotion, vulnerability and searing honesty. With the endless love of her son, the support of her family of friends, Cancer acting as a catalyst and the power of God within, Jacinta unearths an amazing abundance of precious and glorious gifts available to every one of us. Her inspirational story of vulnerability, courage and faith is her gift to you.

A Toxic Beginning

'I don't want to go down here daddy, I am scared'. Daddy looks sad. "You must do as your mother says, Cinty. You will be all right down here. You must stay here until I come back for you and on no account come back upstairs". With tears dropping silently from my eyes, I wave bye bye and clutching my teddy, I slowly clamber down the giant steps. The door shuts suddenly behind me making my little body jump. I know it's my fault, so I have to stay here. I trust Daddy and don't want to get him into trouble with mammy. My little lungs struggle to breathe in the musty, damp air and the dim yet glaring light tortures my tired, tearful eyes. Shivering and terrified, I root myself on top of the heap of rancid coal in the corner away from the ravenous mice scurrying about beneath my ice cold feet. I fully dig out some coal with my hands, trying hard to make a sort of bed for myself, whilst trying to keep my new dress clean or mammy will get angry again. The comforting movement outside the barred window gradually fades as the cruel hand of darkness descends, squeezing the life out of my terrorised little body. I feel alone and responsible for the whole world.

20 April '04 during a follow-up appointment with my GP for HRT, as I am approaching the menopause, my

thorough doctor confirms that my recent womb scan results are fine as I suspected they would be. She goes on to check my blood pressure, acknowledging that it is superb, in fact the best it has ever been! I attribute this to my radical change in career. She then proceeds to check my breasts. Now my left breast has always been bigger than my right. This has never really concerned me especially as I had it checked by the Breast Cancer Consultant at the hospital ten years previously, just after I gave birth to my son Josh. The explanation that I was given then was there was a small cyst 'probably full of water' and a probable result of hormone imbalance due to my age – what a cheek! However, I was relieved. The consultant suggested I take Evening Primrose Oil and Vitamin B12 supplements. This is laughable coming from someone who is inclined to adopt a derisory approach to anything remotely alternative. Looking back, I wish that I had looked into this further, as I now understand that hormone imbalance can be considered (although not proven) as one of the possible contributory causes of Breast Cancer. In fact, this consultant's flippant comments actually gave me a false sense of security about my breast. However, when my doctor feels my left breast, she frowns observing that it feels very lumpy. She immediately fast tracks me to Stoke Mandeville Hospital for a mammogram. This is the start of our life changing experience as a family.

22 April '04 as I do not have a partner as such, I ask my close friend Martin to come with me for the mammogram. As I had an upsetting, uncomfortable experience with an earlier mammogram, I wanted some company and support on this occasion. I am not really concerned

about the results. I feel that my doctor is just taking extra precautions before prescribing HRT. At the hospital, I change into a gown and wait. I am called in quite quickly. I explain to the radiographer what had happened last time and how I am feeling a little nervous this time. I want to make sure that she fully understands how I am feeling and can see me for 'me' and not merely another patient. Although I do not realise it at the time, this is the start of my part in empowering myself through this experience. Something I do as I go along. The radiographer is very understanding and explains the procedure to me before beginning. She then guides me slowly through each stage. Once I know that the radiographer is 'with me', I feel less nervous and not about to be 'done to'. I feel empowered.

Hours pass and suddenly I hear the latch on the door at the top of the cellar steps. Daddy has come for me. I run up the steps with a renewed desperation into daddy's arms. Holding his hand and clutching my teddy, we go back upstairs, my little legs straining to take one stair at a time to keep up with Daddy. He is quiet and looks sad. I hope mammy is not still mad with daddy or me. My insides are all muddled up. I cannot stop shivering. At the top of the stairs, Daddy tells me to go to my room as he solemnly walks back into the kitchen. I wish he would give me a cuddle. I don't know what I have done wrong. I play quietly upstairs alone in my room trying not to make a sound in case I annoy mammy again. I think my brother Gerard and sister Deirdre are in their room playing. I feel left out and not part of what's happening around me. Later, I come down to the kitchen for tea, anxious to see mammy's face. She looks serious but not angry. I take a deep breath and tentatively sit down without so much as a whisper. I am afraid to breathe in case I make everything worse all over again. The terrible stuff has passed for now. That evening we all kneel down as a family amongst the day's smouldering ashes and pray. We say the rosary, pretending the bad things are not that bad.

26 April '04 I wait in reception to see the Consultant. A nurse quickly shows me into the special waiting area. My name is called out and I am shown in to meet the official looking General Consultant. After examining me, he looks at the mammogram results on an illuminated screen, explaining that there are some calcified cells. I ask what this means. His reply changes my world forever: "This is a sign of cancer". This is the first time that I have heard the word cancer. It had not even entered my head before this appointment and, without any time to take this on board, the consultant sits down behind his desk and immediately continues: "You will need a biopsy, I will put your name down. The earliest date we have available is........" I cannot speak or catch my breath. This consultant moves immediately on to the practicalities. I have no time to think or feel. I feel so little all of a sudden and very vulnerable. Don't I have a say in what happens to me? Eventually I manage to blurt out from the depth of my shaken body: "there is a huge difference between my 'needing' a biopsy and my 'deciding if I am going to have one". Immediately the nurse, who has remained silent up to this point, comes to my side and tries to empathise: "you are in shock dear". I feel confused and terrified. I don't know this nurse. I try to explain that I am terrified of needles. Before I can continue, this very professional looking nurse abruptly

interrupts saying that I have a needle phobia, which she promptly adds to my notes. She quickly shows me to the door. I feel dismissed with overwhelming news.

I am in a daze as I wander through reception. The receptionist tells me that I have to go back to the clinic, as I do not have the correct paperwork. Tears silently drop from my eyes. The receptionist gently mentions that it doesn't matter and books me in for my biopsy. I leave the hospital, sit in my car and cry, cry forever.

Why can the consultant not empathise? Is he not human also? It seems to me that the consultant gives the facts and the nurse attempts to give the emotional support! This doesn't work. It is disjointed and too late. Whatever happened to explaining this procedure to me gently, asking how I felt about it and if I was happy about proceeding rather than assuming I will agree? This would have made all the difference.

The glare of the naked light bulb above pierces my sobbing eyes, never leaving me alone. Through the small murky, barred window above, I can see legs of many people walking past on the pavement above, completely unaware of my isolated existence down here. I wish daddy would come to me and take me away from here. Minutes pass painfully slowly blending into long, scary hours, deprived of light and love. What is wrong with me? I don't want to be alone. The fighting upstairs is replaced with sounds of hungry mice down here. I never try to leave because I know daddy will come for me when it is quiet upstairs. As I sit here alone, freezing and frightened, under the piercing, bald light bulb, the raging war upstairs bears down on my small shoulders, deepening my guilt for the problems I have caused.

27 April '04, holding this unbearable news inside me I rush back from a work meeting to pick up my son from school, my mind in turmoil. A speed camera flashes blinding me for a moment capturing me driving at 34 miles per hour. Oh my god, this will bring my total points up to 12. I can't lose my driving licence. How will I get my son to and from school, get myself to radiotherapy eventually in Oxford, attend work meetings around Buckinghamshire and Berkshire. Everything is happening too quickly for me. Having made some calls to my solicitor, I realise quickly that to stand any chance of holding on to my licence, I shall need to present my case myself in court in Oxford. My world is shaking and I am struggling to hold on.

3 May '04 what am I going to do? I am terrified of needles. I cannot face this biopsy under a local anaesthetic. I feel so alone. I telephone the hospital and ask to speak to the Breast Cancer Consultant himself. Surprisingly, he returns my call. I am on my way to work. Hearing my mobile ring, I pull over quickly and stop in a lay-by. I express my deep-rooted fear in absolute detail, hoping he will understand: "Doctor, I was sexually abused as a child and since then I have had a horror of needles. They remind me of my father's abuse". The line goes silent for a few moments, but then he agrees to arrange sedation for me for this procedure. I really appreciate this. I think I can face this procedure, knowing that I shall not be aware of what is happening. I just cannot bear knowing what is happening to me. ....

Read what others say..............

'An inspiring read' by R. Daly
(London, UK) 14 April 2012

I've given this book 5 stars for the author's gutsy determination to be true to herself and to cut the destructive chain of negativity that gets handed down relentlessly, and often totally unquestioned, from generation to generation.

Jacinta is determined that her son should not be another victim of the intense lack of love of which she found herself on the receiving end of. Through being prepared to be ruthlessly honest with, and true to herself, Jacinta slowly identifies the most important ingredients in human relations, and therefore in life – care, empathy, community, a sense of belonging. She shines the light of this understanding on her often inhuman experiences with our British health service as she goes through the rigours of cancer diagnosis and treatment, and contrasts this dramatically with one of the best integrated hospitals in the world, in Mexico, an organisation that has the power to transform her whole experience of life.

By interspersing her journey through cancer with episodes from her childhood, we become acutely aware of how we all, as adults, can become 'damaged goods' unable to respond to life and the people around us in a human and empathic manner, simply because those who brought us into the world and who guide our first steps are themselves 'damaged goods', unaware of the further damage they are wreaking on the next generation by failing to question their lives in the way the author does so courageously.

I hope this book will inspire many more people to find the courage to transform their own lives and to get to the heart of what it means to be a human being – it's desperately needed.

'A moving story', Lynne Stannard – Mason 22 Dec 2013

I found Jacinta's story gripping and very moving. She describes her early life in Derry and the physical and mental torment that she endured, in such a moving manner, that the reader cannot but feel desperately sad for the plight of this lovely little girl.

Her subsequent diagnosis with breast cancer, as a single mother and her incredible strength of spirit and character, plus the tremendous love for her son, takes the story from tragedy through to a higher spiritual awareness and renewed belief.

'Hidden Gifts' is very well worth reading, particularly for those who have suffered abuse, grief or crisis. It is a story of the strength and humour which overcomes the nasty things that life can throw at any of us.

'Engaging, courageous and honest' – Benn

Hidden Gifts may be about cancer and abuse, BUT it is a book about the importance of human spirit and healing. I found Jacinta's story engaging, courageous and honest; not the 'maudlin' approach some might take in a similar position. The journey she makes, she shares; she dwells on her victories and is raw and honest about her fears. I found myself moved as several of my own buttons were pressed. I really appreciated the ways in which Jacinta not only made it obvious there was trauma, but kept it as a significant and blatant undercurrent – that told its own story through the context – without driving pain into the reader. What is striking is how she overcomes these fears, how she releases them and surrenders into healing. Jacinta's story tells of how her cancer healed her intention, her life experience and encouraged her to step into magnificence and self-empowerment.

'An enthralling story' – Ginny

This is an enthralling story of a single mother's journey though breast cancer. Jacinta takes us through her battles with the NHS and their impersonal approach to the holistic and loving environment of the clinic in Mexico where she did her final healing.

The story is written in the present tense, in diary format with flashbacks to her childhood, her terrifying and abusive mother and ineffective and inappropriate father. As Jacinta travels along her path with the breast cancer, the injections and other treatments we see how the past is also healed by coming to the fore..

This is a well written and gripping read that can be enjoyed by everyone, as it is not just about coping with breast cancer but also about being true to oneself and standing up for what one believes in.

'Very moving' – Bogside

I found this to be a very moving book. There were times when I could not put it down and then there were others, so packed with emotion, when I *had* to put it down and take a break. Jacinta McShane's writing style is unstilted and forthright, or perhaps innocent would better describe it. Even though she is not a professional writer, I find that the text flows easily. Her decision to intersperse her fight against cancer as an adult with her childhood memories is very effective and makes the reading more interesting. It also underscores how important are our early experiences in forming who we are as adults.

We see many examples in our society of people who are abused in childhood and who then become abusers themselves later in life. The author is an inspirational counter-example. We can all learn something from her suffering and her successful struggle to become a strong, confident, and loving mother.

'Fascinating and enthralling read' – Dr Russ

I found this book to be a fascinating and enthralling read which is evidenced by the fact that I read it in one go. In it the author chronicles her journey through the distress of the diagnosis and subsequent treatments of her breast cancer and the way in which she fought to remain an individual in a system which finds it easier to detach itself from the person. For this reason alone it would be a useful addition to the reading list of trainee medical personnel.

However, the unique aspect of the author's story is the way in which this trauma enabled her to face up to the demons of a childhood scarred by abuse at home. By means of flashbacks interspersed throughout the narrative, she recalls early years of mistreatment which had remained buried in her psyche, thus stunting a properly rounded development. She explores how her self-denial of the experiences of these early relationships with those who should have provided a loving and secure environment created her own subconscious inadequacies. She goes on to recognise that it is only as a result of accepting what happened as a child that she can now start to enjoy a full, normal life.

The author, therefore, sees her diagnosis as a stimulant to face up to an underlying condition which had to be accepted before it could be addressed. She concludes by explaining how, with the help of her son and her faith, she has started on that road to recovery.

'Positive and uplifting' – Helen 6 Jan 2011
With great clarity and baring of her soul, the author captures the reality of a cancer diagnosis and the rollercoaster journey that follows.

Interspersing it with her childhood experiences adds extra depth and poignancy to the overall uplifting nature of her story.

The discoveries she and her son make show us that valuable lessons can be learned and much heartache and trauma overcome by accepting that dis-ease and disease in our lives must be acknowledged in order to rise above it and live a full life.

As a person on a cancer journey myself, I recommend this book to others in the same position, but also to anyone searching for a positive outlook on life.

'Sensitive' – A. Smith, 10 Nov 2010
This is a book which will be appreciated by people who are interested in people.

It is beautifully and sensitively written, with reflections on the past and the present and making connections between them. It is encouraging to anyone who faces illness, or who feels they are not in control of their life, to take that control and make informed choices.

It is a story of how life can become richer through adversity. A book which will touch the reader.

'A very good read' – Michael, 10 Jun 2011
I thought the book was an amazing story of bravery, courage against the odds and pure determination on both the part of Jacinta and of her son Josh to see it through and come out at the other end better and stronger people as a result.

So often it must be easier to try and deny the bad things that happen and not to deal with the root causes of difficulties, which does affect you in so many ways as you get older, but here is a lady who has overcome and is much better for having done so.

It was very well written and the contrast of the treatment, healing process and the flashback to Jacinta's early years was a good concept and made the reading, albeit hard going at times because if the content, very good.

I know there were dark times for both Jacinta and Josh but through it all the bond between a mother and son is shown as being so very strong.

What I also liked was the way in which it was written also gives hope to others who are going through a similar traumatic time. All the references to the kind and lovely people whose lives are dedicated to helping people in similar situations are there too. Quite often it is who do you turn to or where do you go to get help from, so to have all the references to people and organizations within the book is very good.

The book was made even more real as I have the honour of personally knowing Jacinta and Josh so it meant even more reading it through, both the high and the low parts of the book.